The Doctor's Guide to Chronic Fatigue Syndrome

The Doctor's Guide to Chronic Fatigue Syndrome

Understanding, Treating, and Living with CFIDS

David S. Bell, M.D.

Addison-Wesley Publishing Company
Reading, Massachusetts · Menlo Park, California · New York
Don Mills, Ontario · Wokingham, England · Amsterdam · Bonn
Sydney · Singapore · Tokyo · Madrid · San Juan
Paris · Seoul · Milan · Mexico City · Taipei

12.00

Many of the designations used by manufacturers and sellers to distinguish their products are claimed as trademarks. Where those designations appear in this book and Addison-Wesley was aware of a trademark claim, the designations have been printed in initial capital letters (e.g., Tylenol).

31881710

Library of Congress Cataloging-in-Publication Data

Bell, David S. (David Sheffield)
    The doctor's guide to chronic fatigue syndrome : understanding, treating, and living with CFIDS / David S. Bell.
        p. cm.
    Rev. ed. of: The disease of a thousand names. ©1991.
    Includes bibliographical references and index.
    ISBN 0-201-62616-0
    ISBN 0-201-40797-3 (pbk.)
    1. Chronic fatigue syndrome. I. Bell, David S. (David Sheffield) Disease of a thousand names. II. Title.
    [DNLM: 1. Fatigue Syndrome, Chronic. WC 500 B433db 1993]
RB150.F37B453   1993
616'.047—dc20
DNLM/DLC
for Library of Congress   93-37533
                                                          CIP

65894

RB
150
F37
B453
1995

Cover design by Ned Williams
Text design by Wilson Graphics & Design (Kenneth J. Wilson)
Set in 10-point Palatino by CopyRight, Inc.

1 2 3 4 5 6 7 8 9-DOH-97969594
First printing, December 1993
First paperback printing, December 1994

This book is dedicated in loving memory of

Skye Kristina Dailor
January 28, 1976–September 1, 1990

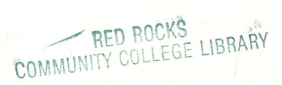

CONTENTS

Alison Williams: A Case History xi

Preface 1

PART 1 **AN OVERVIEW OF CHRONIC FATIGUE
SYNDROME** 5

Chapter 1 **What Is CFIDS?** 7

Symptoms of CFIDS 9
Who Gets CFIDS? 13
Epidemic or Endemic? 14
What Causes CFIDS? 15
The Physician's Dilemma 18

PART 2 **DESCRIPTION OF AN ILLNESS** 23

Chapter 2 **The Course of CFIDS** 25

The Diagnosis 26
Onset—The Turbulent First Six Months 28
Acute Onset? 29
Concept of Trigger Event 31
Clinical Course 32
Symptoms 33
Physical Examination 38
The Neurology of CFIDS 42

Chapter 3 **Could It Be Something Else?** 51

Multiple Sclerosis 51
Depression 52
Somatization and Malingering 56
Biologic Depression 57
Anxiety Disorders 58
Allergies 59

Chemical Sensitivities 62
Fibromyalgia 63
Conclusion 63

Chapter 4 **CFIDS and Children** 65

Kevin Jennings: A Case History 65
A Child's Symptoms 72
School Disorders 76
Emotional Disorders 78
Conclusion 79

PART 3   THE TESTS 81

Chapter 5 **Laboratory Evaluation in CFIDS** 83

Exclusionary Tests 85
More Invasive Tests 89
Conclusion 91

Chapter 6 **The Immunology of CFIDS** 93

Immune System Suppression 94
Immune System Activation 97
Conclusion 102

Chapter 7 **Epstein-Barr Virus** 105

The Debate over EBV Antibodies 107
The Concept of EBV as a Trigger Infection 109
Conclusion 110

Chapter 8 **Research Testing** 111

The Tests 112
Conclusion 117

Chapter 9 **The Measurement of Disability** 119

The Opinion of the Primary Care Physician 120
CFIDS Disability Scale 122
Karnofsky Rating Scale 124
Sickness Impact Profile 125

Kilocalorie Expenditure (Huang and Quinlan Method) 125
Radial Plot of Symptoms 125
Conclusions 130

PART 4 TREATMENT OF CFIDS 133

Chapter 10 **Prognosis or Outcome** 135
Cure Versus Improvement 135
Historical Prognosis 136
Fatal Complications 137
Factors Influencing Recovery 138
Conclusion 143

Chapter 11 **General Treatment Principles** 145
Treatment of Symptoms or Treatment of Underlying Cause? 145
Treatment of Trigger Agent 147
Types of Treatment 148

Chapter 12 **An Approach to Medication** 157
General Principles with Medications 157
The Groups of Medications 159
The Symptom Clusters 164
Conclusion 168

Chapter 13 **What Does the Future Hold?** 169
Treatment Possibilities 169
Conclusion 177

PART 5 THE SEARCH FOR A CAUSE 179

Chapter 14 **The Historical Perspective** 181
CFIDS Epidemics 181
Conclusion 194

Chapter 15 **Theories and Research** 195

One Disease or Many? 195
The Spectrum of Theories 200

Chapter 16 **A Promising Theory** 215

CFIDS and the Flu 215
CFIDS and Cytokines 217
Cytokines and Agent X 219
A CFIDS-Associated Retrovirus? 220
CFIDS and AIDS 222
A Retroviral Cause for CFIDS 226

Conclusions: The Frontier of Twenty-First-Century Medicine 231

Appendices 237

Index 267

Alison Williams
A Case History

It began innocently enough; it was just a case of the "flu." There was some inconvenience because Alison Williams had begun a new job only two months before and was already behind in her work. She was still trying to learn the ropes, but since she was intelligent and creative, it would not be hard. The job—regional sales manager for a small company that was expanding and doing well—was exciting. Alison had a natural ability to work with people, meet deadlines, and find innovative solutions to problems. The "flu" had only complicated her schedule.

She called the office, said she was ill, and went to bed. Her temperature was 101°, and she had a sore throat and swollen lymph nodes; she ached all over. As she swallowed cold tablets, she was reminded of the power of advertising and the natural assumption that these yellow and white pills would make everything better.

Throughout most of the day she slept. Her husband, Ron, was at work and the children were at school, so the house was deserted and quiet. This was really the first day in two months that she had had a chance to rest, and she decided to make the most of it. She wanted to read in the afternoon, but the exhaustion was overwhelming. She would wake, look at the clock, take two aspirin with juice, and sleep again.

The next day Alison awoke without much improvement. She noticed pain in all of her muscles, and her lymph glands were sore as well. She had a headache so severe that she felt her eyes were being pushed out of her head. She still had a fever and resigned herself to another day in bed. She made breakfast and declined her husband's offer to call the doctor. "It's just the flu," she said. "It will pass." She was exhausted, and after the children were on the school bus she went back to bed.

But it didn't pass. Five days later the fever had abated, but pains in her knees and wrists had joined the aching in her muscles. Her eyes ached, and there were episodes of blurred vision. She had spells of light-headedness and dizziness, especially when she sat up or changed position. The headache had not let up during the entire five days. It was now Monday, and her husband had watched the children over the weekend. Alison had an appointment with Dr. Pearson, and she planned to try to go to work afterward.

Dr. Pearson took a brief history and gave her a physical examination. He said her examination was normal, typical of the flu, and that she should be fine within a couple of days. The treatment was bed rest, aspirin, and plenty of liquids. Alison took the aspirin, drank some fluids, and went to work.

Her desk was as messy as when she had left last Wednesday, which was no surprise. Although exhausted, she managed to handle several phone calls and get through a meeting that had been planned long in advance. She had no idea of what was being discussed and was unable to concentrate. After the meeting her boss told her to go home and rest. She looked as if she still had the flu.

Alison's problems continued through the rest of that week. Her thermometer showed that her fever had disappeared, but she felt as if she still had it. Shaking chills and episodes of soaking sweats occurred, frequently at night. Alison spent most of the time in bed and began to take handfuls of vitamin C, advice given to her by her mother. The worst symptom was the exhaustion; the headaches and sore throat were constant, although not as bad. She began having diarrhea, and a skin rash came and went. During the week she slept at least twenty hours a day, but the exhaustion continued. Her back ached from lying in bed so much.

Dr. Pearson ordered a complete blood count, a throat culture for strep, and a "monospot" for infectious mononucleosis because of the persistent sore throat and fatigue. He also did a screening test for hepatitis B because she had joint pains and pain in the liver area on abdominal palpation. All the tests were normal. There had been no recent outbreaks of flu, and he admitted that he did not know why she had not recovered in the twelve days since onset. He prescribed a course of erythromycin, a broad spectrum antibiotic, and hoped that her symptoms would disappear.

During the next week, Alison tried three times to go to work. It was a disaster. Her boss knew her to be honest and hardworking, but it was a sensitive time for the company, and Alison was in an important position with many decisions to be made. One of her colleagues was appointed temporary sales manager, so at least the pressure was off. Perhaps there had been too much stress. Alison could now relax and concentrate on getting well.

But concentrating—indeed, any kind of thinking—had become very difficult. At first she attributed it to the exhaustion, but it was more than that. She had tried to read a sales projection report, something so familiar to her that she could have written it herself. But she was unable to make it through the first paragraph without becoming lost. Her eyes had difficulty focusing on the words, and her mind seemed unable to digest more than three words at a time. Reading had become impossible—her eyes saw the words on the page, but she could make no sense of them.

The fatigue continued. She had been ill now for almost three weeks and could stay up for about half the day. She cooked the family meals, but the slightest activity left her breathless with exhaustion. She had never felt like this before, although she had had the flu several times. Clearly, this was no ordinary flu.

Dr. Pearson expressed concern that she was not recovering, but he had no answers other than that this must be a viral infection. He ordered a chest X ray and a battery of blood tests, but again no abnormality was found. Aside from tenderness in the lymph glands, muscles, and abdomen, nothing was abnormal on physical examination. She said she felt poorly, but the tests said she should be feeling well. Because of the abdominal pain and diarrhea, Dr. Pearson ordered an upper and lower gastrointestinal series of tests. Alison suspected that they would be normal, and they were.

Alison now became concerned that the symptoms might be due to a hidden malignancy. She remembered that her grandmother had been ill for three months before they found cancer in her pancreas. Her grandmother died soon afterward. Dr. Pearson would not lie to her about something like this, but he was probably just not able to find it. There was something definitely wrong; she felt as if she were dying.

Her husband had been extremely supportive and helpful during this time. They had a good marriage and were able to communicate well. But Ron also had begun to suspect that something was terribly wrong. The flu shouldn't continue for three weeks, no matter what Dr. Pearson said. Ron had noticed Alison's waking during the night with soaking sweats and chills, and she had never before had the flushing rash on her cheeks that was so prominent now. He tried to act as if he believed that everything would be fine, but Alison knew he was worried.

About a week later, after trying several times to reach Dr. Pearson, Ron finally got through. The doctor suggested a consultation with an infectious disease specialist in a nearby city, and an appointment was made for two weeks later. If Alison recovered by then, the appointment could always be canceled. The consultation would be expensive, but there was no alternative. At least the Williamses had good insurance coverage.

Two weeks later, Alison felt a little improved but not well enough to return to work. She had been put on temporary disability by her company, although they had difficulty putting "the flu" down as the diagnosis. She continued to have daily headaches over her eyes and had developed a second type of headache, one of pressure in the back of the head. Alison, in an attempt to keep up her good humor, joked with her husband that she was becoming a connoisseur of headaches, and she preferred the frontal headache to the pressure headache any day.

The sore throat continued as well as the pain in the lymph glands in her neck. She also noticed tender lumps in her armpits, which she had forgotten to tell Dr. Pearson about during her last visit. Her muscles and joints hurt, but there was no obvious swelling in the joints. The stomach pains continued, even worsening somewhat, while the other symptoms had improved. But the exhaustion continued unchanged. Every day, it was as if she had not slept at all; she was as tired after twelve hours of sleep as she had been the day before.

Alison still could not read. It seemed to make the headaches worse, and nothing she tried to read made any sense. Worse yet, she noticed that her memory was not as good as it had been. She wanted to call her secretary at the office in an attempt to stay in touch, but she could not remember her secretary's name. She could not remember the office telephone number. She had always been proud of her excellent memory, but now she had to write down the phone number before she could call.

It was around this time that she became aware that she could walk into a room and not be able to remember what she had come for. Her husband joked that she was losing her marbles, and immediately regretted saying it. By this time Alison was looking a little better; aside from the occasional rash on her cheeks, there was no obvious change from five weeks earlier. She had lost ten pounds because of the diarrhea and lack of appetite.

She had been ill for six weeks when she saw the infectious disease specialist. Ron took the day off from work, and they arrived early for the appointment. Alison was exhausted and was having a "bad" day, which was good because the specialist could see her at her worst. The wall across from her was covered with diplomas and awards, attesting to the idea that there must be nothing this doctor didn't know.

The interview lasted twenty minutes, the physical examination ten minutes more. By the end, the specialist did not seem particularly impressed with Alison. In fact, he acted disappointed, as if he had hoped to find an enormous abscess and it wasn't there. Alison felt as if she had somehow failed the examination. She felt as sick as ever but didn't look sick enough. The infectious disease specialist ordered several more tests, including a CT scan (a computerized X ray) of the brain and more blood work, in an effort to find any unusual infection such as cytomegalovirus, toxoplasmosis, or Lyme disease, none of which Alison and Ron had ever heard of. If one was causing the problem, the physician would explain it to them, but not now.

Two weeks later they returned and learned that the tests were normal. The specialist asked a few questions about how she was feeling, but did not seem to hear when she said that she felt as ill as ever. He did a brief physical examination, which appeared to be a waste of time, and asked Ron if his wife was under any unusual stress. Ron answered that she hadn't been prior to the illness. The specialist suggested that she have a psychiatric interview, since fatigue is a prominent symptom of depression. He felt that depression was probably causing all the symptoms. Alison and Ron were stunned. They returned home without speaking, and later agreed that they felt the infectious disease specialist was nuts.

The fatigue continued, and Alison noticed a few new symptoms: occasionally her heart started racing, and one day she had several episodes of shortness of breath. Dr. Pearson ordered an electrocardiogram and another chest X ray, which again were normal. An echocardiogram showed a mild prolapse of the mitral valve, and he prescribed propranolol, a medication to control the rate of the heartbeat. This medication was also used for migraine, and it was hoped that it might help with Alison's headaches. The rapid heartbeat improved, but the fatigue became worse, so Alison cut the dosage in half without telling Dr. Pearson.

Alison had been very disturbed by the suggestion that she was depressed, yet she decided to consider it. Before the illness, her life had been going in the right direction. She had two wonderful children and a husband who loved her. She had been succeeding at work, although she was now in danger of losing her job. She had to admit it, she was now depressed. She was beginning to think the specialist was right.

They decided to get a second opinion from another infectious disease specialist. This time Alison emphasized the pain in her lymph nodes and the fact that she had been happy and well adjusted before getting the "flu." The specialist concentrated on the lymph nodes more carefully and noted that they were somewhat swollen, although not dramatically. He repeated the routine blood tests and also included tests for AIDS, lupus, rheumatoid arthritis, and thyroid disease. At the end of the visit, the specialist suggested a lymph node biopsy.

The biopsy, on a node in her left armpit, was arranged with a local surgeon and would be performed under general anesthesia. Ron and Alison reported to the hospital at 7 A.M. and went through the usual routines for outpatient surgery. They would be home in three hours. The surgery was uneventful, and the surgeon reported to Ron that there had been no problems. They removed a one-centimeter node from the left axillary region and sent it for complete analysis, including tests for lymphoma and other types of cancer.

Alison had great difficulty recovering from the anesthesia. Two hours after emerging from the operating room she was so groggy that she could not sit up, and her discharge from the hospital was delayed. Six hours later she felt severely ill and was admitted to the surgical floor for observation. Her heartbeat was rapid and her blood pressure was low, but not dangerously. Her headache was severe, and the sore throat returned, probably because of the tube used during surgery. But the exhaustion was the biggest problem. Unable to sit up without becoming dizzy, she slept for the next ten hours. She was as ill now as she had been at the beginning of the illness ten weeks ago.

Alison stayed in the hospital for two days and had not improved much when she finally did go home. There was no change for the next three weeks; she was confined to bed because of an illness that no one could identify and some doubted even existed.

Then she received a notice that her insurance company would not pay for the hospitalization because it had not been necessary following such a minor surgical procedure. The unnecessary hospitalization cost $538, but at least the cost of the biopsy was covered.

The biopsy was normal. There was no lymphoma, and the swelling was due to "reactive hyperplasia," a term pathologists use when nothing much shows up. They cultured the node for bacteria, viruses, fungi, and tuberculosis, none of which was found. Alison showed no emotion when the second infectious disease specialist suggested that she see a counselor about her persistent fatigue.

"This seems like a bad dream," Alison thought as she prepared for work the next day. If there was nothing wrong with her, she could work; maybe working would "shake it out of her." At the office, she felt like a stranger. Things had changed since she had been there last, and she did not know where to start. Although she felt exhausted and had a severe headache, she was determined to work despite it. She was able to go through certain routines but was unable to do anything productive. She realized that in order to pick up where she had left off, she would have to be sharp, to apply her keen mind to the business details, and this she was completely unable to do. Her mind would not function. She was able to control her body to sit at her desk, but the lethargy, exhaustion, and pain made her useless. She felt lost, a stranger in the office where she had once been boss. She could not remember the names of most of the people. At noon she went home, now truly depressed.

She saw Dr. Pearson in his office. They had always been on good terms, and Alison knew him to be honest and straightforward. "Do you think that all these symptoms are due to depression?" she asked him.

"I really have no idea of what is wrong," he answered, obviously uncomfortable. "As you know, the specialists you saw suggested that you see a psychiatrist, and I assume that they are attributing your symptoms to depression. At first I didn't think that depression was causing your symptoms, but now I am not so sure. You look very depressed to me now."

"I am depressed now," Alison answered, "but I wasn't four months ago when all this began."

There was a pause, and Dr. Pearson seemed to agree with what she had said. "I don't know what is wrong," he said, "and depression is one possibility that we haven't really looked into. If I could think of any other possibility, I would be happy to explore it.

Perhaps it would be a good idea to see Dr. Jennings, whom I know to be an excellent psychiatrist." Dr. Pearson did not schedule any further follow-up visits.

Alison agreed, and an appointment was set up. It seemed to her that Dr. Pearson had suggested she see Dr. Jennings mainly because he didn't know what to do with her, and he wanted her off his back. Maybe that was a little harsh. After all, he had been honest and admitted that he didn't think she was nuts. Alison's thinking was not clear, but she felt she understood one message: Dr. Pearson didn't know what was wrong, but didn't want to see her anymore. Alison had become a nuisance to him.

The months began to fade into one another, holidays came and went; seasons blended into a confusing array of different weather patterns. Alison lost her job, and the disability payments stopped. Once she had thought of herself as a creative, energetic woman, capable of a full-time job, capable of being a full-time mother and a full-time wife. There had been no doubt, no hesitation. Life offered opportunities and happiness.

Now she was a dependent invalid, unable to leave her house and spending most of her days in bed. She had lost the enjoyment of her children and her home. She had lost the joys of family activities, shopping, even cooking. But worst of all, she had lost her self-confidence: was she sick or just crazy? She knew nothing now, neither telephone numbers nor who she really was. She could read words but could not follow the directions of a cookbook. She could not drive because she would get lost in the neighborhood. Yet the doctors kept telling her that nothing was seriously wrong.

Even the tests seemed to come and go. She went to a neurologist who did a lumbar puncture, an MRI (magnetic resonance imaging) scan of the brain, muscle biopsies, a liver biopsy, more blood tests. None of the tests was abnormal. Doxepin, an antidepressant medication, was prescribed at the usual doses, and she felt even more exhausted. When the dosage was reduced to one appropriate for a child, she felt a little better.

But overwhelming problems remained. Alison persisted with weekly visits to the psychiatrist, but nothing much seemed to be happening. She really didn't know if the psychiatrist had any idea of what was wrong. Every time she asked his opinion, he just said she was depressed.

Of course, she had to agree with him. She had begun thinking of suicide recently, not so much for herself as to ease the burden on her family. She saw herself sliding down an endless hillside, about to plunge into an abyss. She thought she was dying, and now wanted it to end quickly. Nothing made sense anymore. She suspected that even Ron was thinking she was crazy. They were not talking the way they used to, and he was always taking the children out somewhere to make the house quiet. She didn't know if he was trying to make her more comfortable or hide her from the children.

New symptoms appeared. Among the most disturbing was numbness in her legs, a symptom the neurologist thought could be due to multiple sclerosis. But the tests did not confirm MS. She also developed ringing in her ears, balance problems, and occasional double vision. The ophthalmologist could give no explanation. Her speech and handwriting were both affected. The muscles in her right arm clearly appeared weaker than previously, something the neurologist attributed to atrophy. But there was no explanation of why there should be atrophy in the first place.

All of these new symptoms were added to the original ones, which had not disappeared. Worst of all was the exhaustion, the fatigue. It was now better than in the first few months of the illness, or had she just become more used to it? The headaches continued, usually in the front over her eyes, but occasionally also as pressure in the back of her skull, as if her head would explode. The sore throats were less frequent, but the joint pains was worse. The pain in her muscles and lymph nodes remained about the same. Almost every night she would awake with drenching sweats.

Alison developed insomnia, despite the severe fatigue. Although exhausted, she would lie in bed unable to sleep. Her muscles would twitch and she could not become comfortable. If she did fall asleep, she would awake after a few hours, often with the sweats. She took sleeping pills, and although they helped somewhat, it was not enough to make her comfortable. Alison was pale, except when she had that flushing of her cheeks. She stopped going to the psychiatrist.

About eighteen months after first becoming ill, Alison began to feel better. The symptoms were still present, but they were milder and she was used to them now. She could plan activities, knowing what would make her feel sick and what she could tolerate. She could go shopping with the children, although she knew it meant that she would have to stay in bed the next day. But it was worth it. She kept to a very strict diet, having learned that certain foods made her feel worse. Alcohol usually made her feel sick, and she had long ago given that up. Even her thinking was improving. She could only hope that it would continue. She stopped talking about her symptoms and very rarely visited physicians.

But she had never really gained back her self-confidence. She avoided doctors, and when she saw one she would not bring up the exhaustion or the pains. She did not dare to expose herself to what she perceived as the inevitable diagnosis of hypochondria. Alison assumed that the physicians thought she was just trying to get sympathy. She gave up trying to obtain disability payments, for after the first rejection she felt she did not have the strength to fight. How could she prove that she was really sick? All the tests were normal, and only the test results seemed to count.

It was around this time that she heard of chronic fatigue / immune dysfunction syndrome (CFIDS), and that it might be related to the virus that causes infectious mononucleosis. She saw Dr. Pearson and asked for a test of the Epstein-Barr virus, on the chance that it might be "chronic mono." Although not familiar with the syndrome, he ordered the test and was surprised to find that the results did not fit the pattern of either new or old infection, yet they were abnormal. After eighteen months and over $15,000 in medical tests, Alison finally had one that was abnormal.

Finding this abnormal test, which implied a "reactivation" of the Epstein-Barr virus in her system, did nothing to improve her symptoms. She still had no medication that would cure her. She later learned that the Epstein-Barr virus antibody was not even a good test for CFIDS. But it did resolve an issue that was destroying her life almost as much as the symptoms themselves: she was not a hypochondriac. Perhaps she had known it all along, but she had needed this confirmation to regain her lost self-confidence. Her self-esteem had been just as sick as her body. Now she would begin the process of healing her dignity.

PREFACE

When physicians know very little about an illness, they often attempt to disguise their lack of knowledge by using a variety of names for the disease. The number of names is inversely proportional to the amount of knowledge. Certainly this is true of chronic fatigue syndrome.

Chronic fatigue syndrome (CFS) is one of a multitude of names for a poorly understood illness that has finally begun to gain long-deserved attention. The confusion, controversy, and misunderstandings surrounding this illness have led directly to an increased burden of suffering for those who have it. Although "chronic fatigue syndrome" is the term most frequently used by medical specialists, it is often confused with the generic symptom of "chronic fatigue." A recent article in a prominent medical journal made this common mistake, adding to the confusion among health professionals.

Many illnesses, such as diabetes, cancer, anxiety, and depression, can cause the symptom of chronic fatigue. However, chronic fatigue *syndrome* is distinct from the multitude of fatigue-causing illnesses; it is a specific constellation of symptoms—a unique syndrome. I therefore prefer to use the term "chronic fatigue / immune dysfunction syndrome" (CFIDS), since it combines the symptom of fatigue with the presence of immune system markers, thus separating it from generic chronic fatigue.

The first edition of this book was titled *The Disease of a Thousand Names*, and some of the many names are presented in chapter one and the chapter on CFIDS history. Although some of the name confusion has begun to abate, it has by no means disappeared. It is very likely that when the cause of CFIDS becomes understood, the useless controversy over the name will finally come to rest. I hope that time will soon be at hand.

At the time of this writing, the medical profession has remained largely uninformed about the newer developments in CFIDS research. Indeed, many physicians seem to still be debating whether the illness exists at all. It is tragically ironic that the public, mostly due to the efforts of the many support groups for CFIDS, is far more aware and informed of this common disease than are physicians. The purpose of this book is to provide an overview of the current knowledge of CFIDS, including its history, signs and symptoms, clinical course, laboratory findings, and the recent advances. In addition, research concerning possible causes will be described. General principles of symptomatic treatment will be discussed, along with directions for the future. References to published articles will be given for those wishing to pursue this topic in greater depth.

This book is meant for only general education on CFIDS, and should not be considered a medical text. It was written for people with CFIDS or those who have some interest in the illness. I hope that it will provide an introduction for practicing physicians and a starting point for further study. An attempt has been made to simplify the medical issues, and any simplification necessarily adds distortion. For those readers who may have CFIDS, this book is in no way meant to replace medical care, and any general suggestions should be checked with your own physician, as your circumstances and even diagnosis may be quite different.

I freely admit to bias in writing this book. I fully believe that CFIDS is a specific, organic illness, caused by a specific agent or agents. I make no claims to be impartial in the argument of whether or not the illness is real. It is interesting that among researchers directly involved in epidemics of CFIDS, there is no discussion of this question. Personal experience has made the issue irrelevant and even insulting.

There are many to whom I am indebted in the writing of this book. I could name fifty researchers whom I consider close friends and who have freely taught me about CFIDS. The open sharing of research data and ideas in CFIDS has been remarkable, perhaps greater than has occurred in relation to any other illness. We may be witnessing a new era in which research cooperation has replaced competition. The information in this book has either been published or presented at scientific meetings, except for a few instances where unreported data have been used with permission.

I am indebted to the CFIDS support groups for their unending enthusiasm and encouragement. I am forever in the debt of my research assistants Jean Pollard, Paula Corser, and Cathie Barry, without whose help I would not have begun to approach the subject. I would like to thank Nancy Weaver, Kathy Grigg, Marc Iverson, and many others for their help and support. The Lyndonville Area Foundation is probably the first organization in the United States to have helped with the financial burden of studying CFIDS, and they did so out of a desire to help the people of Lyndonville, New York, and without expectation of financial return. Again it is a sign of a new era; local community organizations, support groups, and individuals have funded medical research while federal agencies did little. But my greatest thanks is to the many patients who have taught me about CFIDS. My hope is that someday their kindness and patience in the face of suffering will be repaid by effective treatments for those with continuing symptoms and by prevention of this illness for those yet to become ill.

It is also my hope that this book will soon be obsolete. I hope for new discoveries that will answer the many questions posed in these pages. Medical research has met some early goals in studying this illness, establishing it as a major public health threat of the 1990s. The progress during this time, however, has been agonizingly slow, an era that I hope has passed. But even if new information soon outdates the speculations offered in this book, the clinical details, the symptoms, and basic laboratory findings should remain of some value.

We still know little about this illness. The ideas contained in this book need to be confirmed by slow, methodical, and accurate scientific research. It is possible that we are standing at the door of major medical breakthroughs, and that CFIDS is the key. I have no doubt that with the understanding of this illness will also come understanding of numerous other conditions—and an end to the absurd argument of whether this illness is real, an unnecessary argument that has caused so much pain and added so greatly to the burden of those ill with chronic fatigue / immune dysfunction syndrome.

David S. Bell, M.D.
Cambridge, Massachusetts, 1993

PART 1

An Overview of Chronic Fatigue Syndrome

CHAPTER 1

What Is CFIDS?

*A*lison Williams's battle with chronic fatigue / immune dysfunction syndrome (CFIDS) is a fictional account, yet it is typical of thousands of people. What is this strange illness? Who gets it? Why has it been so hard to pin down? Is it new? What causes it? This chapter will take a broad look at these questions before we delve into the intricacies of this devastating illness.

CFIDS ("see-fids") is one of about fifty names for an illness that only recently has become recognized as a specific entity. The illness has been called chronic Epstein-Barr virus syndrome (CEBV), post-viral fatigue syndrome (PVFS), and chronic mononucleosis. It has been ridiculed and demeaned with the term "yuppie flu." In Great Britain, Australia, New Zealand, and many other parts of the world it is called myalgic encephalomyelitis (ME). It is possible that this illness is the same as or closely related to fibromyalgia. "Chronic fatigue / immune dysfunction syndrome" is perhaps the most widely known name in the United States and is synonymous with the term "chronic fatigue syndrome" (CFS). The list keeps growing.

The name "chronic fatigue syndrome" was proposed in 1988 by the Centers for Disease Control in a paper describing the diagnostic criteria (Holmes 88), and much of the recent research in this country uses it. I think that few people, especially patients, really like the term. It implies a benign condition of almost no importance in which people are tired, maybe bored, probably because they work too hard or are depressed. But it has become obvious that CFIDS is not a minor or benign illness due to the stresses and strains of daily life. It is a serious, debilitating disease that robs its victims of both their health and their dignity.

In this book I have chosen to use the name "chronic fatigue / immune dysfunction syndrome," or CFIDS, because it combines the most prominent symptom, fatigue, with the presence of a dysfunctional immune system. The name is designed to separate the illness from the chronic fatigue caused by the stresses of daily life. However, the name of the illness is not as important as its understanding, and I am equally at home with almost all other names. I like the term "myalgic encephalomyelitis" used in the United Kingdom; it is a little harsh and somewhat technical, but there can be no doubt that it represents a real disease. It sounds as if it could be fatal. My personal favorite has always been the "Tapanui flu." Each of the many names used to describe this illness has its own history, some describing the illness by the location where it was noted, some attempting to define one or more prominent symptoms. But probably none of the present names will survive; when the cause of the illness is understood, the name will change once again.

To see CFIDS as a reproducible set of symptoms is to recognize its existence, and this is one of the many areas of controversy that have surrounded the illness for the past twenty years. The argument over what causes CFIDS could rage for another twenty years, and probably will, but its existence as a syndrome has been established by the Centers for Disease Control. This somewhat limited advance comes as a starting point for research and as welcome news to patients left without answers.

CFIDS can be defined relatively simply: it is an illness characterized by months or years of severe exhaustion and pain in nearly every part of the body. It has many symptoms, perhaps as many as forty, and each patient may have a slightly different combination of these symptoms. Some physicians, baffled by severe functional limitation and lengthy lists of symptoms while seeing only minimal abnormalities on physical examination, have been unwilling to recognize CFIDS as a syndrome. Many have reacted by suspecting emotional disease or, worse, malingering. But the basic pattern of these symptoms is the same from person to person, and it is this pattern that establishes it as a syndrome.

An illness with fifty names and almost as many symptoms? There are possibly as many theories about its cause as there are names to describe it. The chapters that follow will attempt to sort out the basic issues and tie them together with a cohesive theory.

*S*ymptoms *of* CFIDS

The nonspecific nature of the name CFIDS is appropriate because while there are many symptoms, disabling fatigue and exhaustion are the most prominent and consistent. However, fatigue, probably the most universal symptom, is the most severe symptom in only half of the patients. The rest have either headaches, muscle pain, joint pain, visual disturbances, emotional changes, memory loss, confusion, lymph node pain, or abdominal pain as the most severe symptom. Individual symptoms may vary in intensity, but the pattern of symptoms remains remarkably constant. These symptoms can be completely disabling and may persist for years, or they may be minor to the degree of being no more than a nuisance.

In general, the physical examination shows only subtle abnormalities, such as throat inflammation or muscle and lymph node tenderness. It is truly remarkable that a patient can feel so bad yet look relatively well. The routine laboratory evaluation, like the physical examination, shows only minimal, if any, abnormalities. Although sophisticated laboratory testing may reveal abnormal results, they are difficult for most physicians to interpret and have been largely ignored. The combination of numerous severe somatic complaints and only minor abnormalities on physical exam and routine laboratory testing is the reason many physicians have dismissed this illness as hypochondriasis.

In the past fifty years, the emphasis in medicine has been to divide illnesses into categories by the nature of the symptoms. Therefore, a joint specialist would see CFIDS as a form of arthritis, a psychiatrist would see it as mental illness, and an allergist would see it as a manifestation of allergies. It is ironic that in this day of specialists, the generalists have been the only group of physicians able to recognize the spectrum of symptoms in CFIDS as a specific syndrome. But in our era of technology, it is rare for specialists to listen to generalists.

And specialists have been unable to make much progress in studying this illness, primarily because of the lack of "disease" in the organs in which they specialize. That is to say, although the muscles hurt, muscle biopsies are normal or show minimal changes only. Although there are headaches, CT scans of the brain are normal. Specialists are interested in diseases originating in their area of specialty. In these days of specialty medicine, a patient with CFIDS might see more than ten different specialists, and none will be able to find the cause of the complaints. In CFIDS, whatever causes the symptoms is outside of the limited specialties. We are witnessing a disease so fundamental in its origin that it affects all body systems but causes little damage.

Following is a list of the myriad symptoms seen in CFIDS, including a rough estimate of the percentage of patients who would have each symptom. Those symptoms that cause patients the greatest discomfort are asterisked (*).

*Fatigue or exhaustion	95%
*Headache	90%
*Malaise	80%
*Short-term memory loss	80%
*Muscle pain	75%
*Difficulty concentrating	70%
*Joint pain	65%
*Depression	65%
*Abdominal pain	60%
*Lymph node pain	50%
*Sore throat	50%
*Lack of restful sleep	90%
Muscle weakness	30%
Bitter or metallic taste	25%
Balance disturbance	30%

Diarrhea	50%
Constipation	40%
Bloating	60%
Panic attacks	30%
Eye pain	30%
Scratchiness in eyes	60%
Blurring of vision	80%
Double vision	10%
Sensitivity to bright lights	80%
Numbness and/or tingling in extremities	60%
Fainting spells	40%
Light-headedness	75%
Dizziness	30%
Clumsiness	30%
Insomnia	65%
Fever or sensation of fever	85%
Chills	30%
Night sweats	50%
Weight gain	40%
Allergies	60%
Chemical sensitivities	25%
Palpitations	55%
Shortness of breath	30%
Flushing rash of the face and cheeks	40%
Swelling of the extremities or eyelids	20%
Burning on urination	20%
Sexual dysfunction	20%
Hair loss	20%

A list of CFIDS symptoms is misleading. At first glance it appears that almost every symptom possible is part of the list. This is another reason many physicians have not accepted the reality of CFIDS—there are simply too many symptoms. But a patient relating these symptoms does not list them in a random manner. They fit a precise pattern that is nearly identical from one patient to the next. The pattern of symptoms is so reproducible in the usual case that patients are able to diagnose CFIDS in others in an instant.

Historically, the pattern of symptoms has made the diagnosis of an illness. For example, a patient with fever, malaise, exhaustion, pain in the upper right side of the abdomen, dark urine, light-colored stools, and yellow skin has hepatitis. The precise combination of symptoms is remarkably similar from patient to patient. It is necessary to check the size of the liver and measure liver enzymes to confirm the diagnosis, but the clinical impression, not the laboratory, establishes the diagnosis.

Physicians seeing a patient with CFIDS have been unable or unwilling to recognize a pattern of symptoms, thus questioning the existence of the illness. Perhaps it is because CFIDS is new and we are just not familiar enough with it. Or maybe there are so many symptoms that few physicians are willing to take a full hour to listen to them. Perhaps any mention of an unfamiliar pattern triggers a Pavlovian response diagnosis of depression, a catchall or wastepaper-basket diagnosis for everything poorly understood. And, in defense of my colleagues, on first hearing, this pattern of symptoms seems to make no sense whatsoever.

Another reason some physicians have been reluctant to consider CFIDS as a real disease is the commonplace nature of many of the symptoms. Who has not felt tired, even exhausted, at times? Everyone has headaches now and then, everyone gets an upset stomach. There is nothing special about a sore throat or even muscle aches. Diarrhea, nervousness, depression—all are part of daily life. But CFIDS is not just numerous isolated minor complaints. It is exhaustion that can be incapacitating, severe daily headaches—the diagnosis is made by the presence of these symptoms with a severity that totally disrupts a person's life.

The entire spectrum of CFIDS severity is not known. It is possible that many people have it in a mild form with just a little fatigue, a few too many headaches, a little too much abdominal pain. But the diagnosis of CFIDS at the present time requires a major reduction in activity. It is common to hear patients state that they have been able to function at only half strength for the past three years.

If someone is functioning normally with these symptoms, he or she may indeed have a mild form of CFIDS, but I would not make the diagnosis.

At the time of this writing, CFIDS is still officially considered to be a diagnosis of exclusion. That is, the diagnosis can be considered only when all other diseases that can cause these symptom clusters are eliminated from consideration. In other words, a patient has CFIDS if you don't know what is wrong. This approach, the diagnosis by exclusion, is inappropriate.

It is true that a patient with hypothyroidism can be fatigued, and a patient with a brain tumor can have headaches. Therefore, as in any medical evaluation, other diseases need to be considered and excluded by appropriate testing if the symptom pattern and severity are suggestive. But this approach can be difficult in CFIDS because there are so many illnesses that share some of these symptoms. In general, those common illnesses suggested by the patient's symptoms need to be ruled out. But the uniqueness of the pattern of symptoms in CFIDS, and their persistence over long periods of time, make this an illness that can be diagnosed clinically, not just resorted to when everything else has been excluded.

At the turn of the century, Sir William Osler said about syphilis, "To understand syphilis is to understand all of medicine." I cannot think of a better description of CFIDS. Virtually every organ system is involved, and the clinician needs to look not only at the specific organ systems but to the functioning of the patient as a whole.

*W*ho Gets CFIDS?

The term "yuppie flu" was coined in 1985 to describe sufferers of CFIDS in an epidemic in Incline Village, Nevada. The area was relatively affluent, so CFIDS was designated an illness of the young and affluent. An associated implication was that the illness was trivial and related to being rich and bored and living a yuppie lifestyle. This unfortunate misunderstanding has caused great suffering in patients who have not been taken seriously because of it.

Who does get CFIDS? Only preliminary answers can be offered at present. In epidemics occurring in communities, the majority of patients are adults, although 30 percent are children. But the lack of an objective marker of the illness makes statistics unreliable. Children may be more likely to improve. They also may receive less attention than adults. Of the children affected, boys and girls have the illness with almost equal frequency. The illness is rare under the age of five.

Among adults, women appear to develop the illness more frequently than men. This is true of several immunological diseases, such as lupus erythematosis or rheumatoid arthritis. Estimates are that 60 to 70 percent of adults with CFIDS are women. The most common age range is from twenty to forty, but all ages are affected.

I do not believe that economics or lifestyles are factors in who develops CFIDS. Poor patients certainly get the illness, but they may be less likely to confront their physicians when they are not satisfied with symptom explanations. They do not have economic resources to persist with their doctor until adequate evaluations are done. I suspect that CFIDS may be a major contributor to the homeless problem in this country, a suspicion that may require years to be tested.

*E*pidemic or Endemic?

CFIDS occurs all over the world. At least fifty outbreaks have been recorded in the world's literature—in cities, rural areas, developed countries, and Third World countries. The illness may occur sporadically or in discrete epidemics. As a sporadic illness it is difficult to recognize, but in an epidemic the repetitive nature of the symptoms becomes obvious. In a given community there may be two to ten cases a year. In an epidemic, as occurred in Iceland in 1950, there were 1,100 cases over two years. The epidemiology of these epidemics imply an infectious cause, but one of the great questions surrounding this mysterious illness is whether the infectious agent is the true cause of CFIDS or merely a trigger that causes the illness to appear.

What Causes CFIDS?

The cause of chronic fatigue / immune dysfunction syndrome is not known, but it is probably caused by immune system dysfunction. The symptoms are caused not by something injuring the body, but by the body trying to protect itself from something. It is similar in concept to allergies: the symptoms of allergies are due to the body trying to protect itself from something relatively harmless, such as ragweed pollen. Let us call the underlying cause of CFIDS, whatever it may turn out to be, Agent X. This Agent X probably causes the body little problem in itself, but the immune system overreacts to it, causing severe symptoms.

One reason CFIDS has been so long in gaining acceptance is that it does not fit the model of most infectious diseases. By itself, Agent X causes little or no tissue damage, the markers that physicians traditionally look for. If you suspect someone has been shot, you look for a bullet hole. There is no simple bullet hole in patients with CFIDS. The error that physicians have made is to assume that because there is no visible bullet hole, the patient is not sick. Let us examine several models of illness and look at them in light of what we know about CFIDS.

Mechanical Damage Model

In this model an organ of the body is injured by mechanical means. A car accident is a good example. Let us presume that a patient is in a car accident and the steering wheel is pressed against the liver, causing damage. The diagnosis is straightforward. There is pain in the liver area, the liver is enlarged because of bleeding and inflammation, and blood tests indicate that the liver tissue is not working properly. The symptoms are consistent with liver injury. Furthermore, the symptoms resolve in the expected time with the normal healing process.

This model, which obviously does not fit CFIDS, is one reason physicians have been reluctant to accept CFIDS as a real disease. Although a patient frequently has a history of a precipitating event (such as a car accident), the event can be as diverse as a viral infection or emotional stress. Some patients have no clear event at all;

there is pain, but no physical abnormality or biochemical change typical of damage to the liver, lung, or other "conventional" organs. There is loss of function of the whole being, but no loss of function in any specific organ. Everything seems to hurt, but tests of organ function show no abnormalities. The mechanical damage model does not work (Figure 1–1).

Infectious Disease Model

This model is closely allied to the mechanical damage model, but instead of a car accident there is an infection that is limited to a specific organ system. Take, for example, an infection caused by the hepatitis A virus, one of the most common causes of hepatitis.

This model, shown in Figure 1–2, is the same as the mechanical damage model except that instead of being involved in a car accident, the patient has been spending time with a cousin who has hepatitis. In addition to pain, there are other typical symptoms of liver disease, such as jaundice, white stools, dark urine, and fever. Through physical examination and the measuring of elevated liver enzymes, injury to the liver can be determined. The infectious disease model, like the mechanical damage model, is inadequate for explaining CFIDS, and for the same reasons.

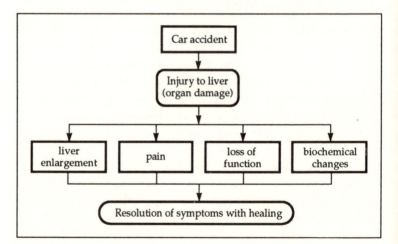

Figure 1–1

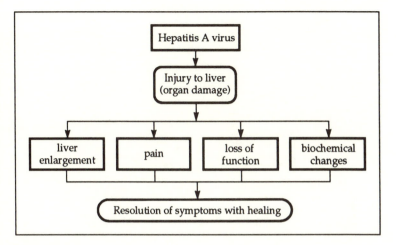

Figure 1–2

Immune Reaction Model

In this model, illness is produced by the body's response to an insult rather than by a direct injury to an organ system. Examples of immune reaction diseases include common allergies, glomerulonephritis, rheumatic fever, lupus erythematosis, and possibly multiple sclerosis. In this model, shown in Figure 1–3, the immune system, in one of many possible ways it can react, responds to ragweed pollen as a threat and mounts an attack against it. It causes mast cells to release histamine, which causes the stuffy nose, sneezing, hives, and other symptoms associated with allergies. The disease is caused not by ragweed pollen but by the body's reaction to it.

Although not commonly thought of as an immune reaction disease, infectious mononucleosis is an excellent example of an illness with symptoms that result from the attempt to fight the virus or viruses that cause it. Several different agents can cause infectious mononucleosis, the Epstein-Barr virus being perhaps the best known.

The parallels in the history of the recognition of AIDS as a specific disease and the recognition of CFIDS are remarkable. For

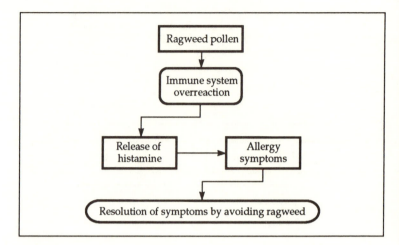

Figure 1–3

years physicians and health care administrators said that no illness could explain fatigue, weight loss, lymph node cancer, unusual parasitic pneumonias, and the purple spots of Kaposi's sarcoma. Because patients with AIDS were dying, it was finally and somewhat reluctantly agreed that this constellation of unusual symptoms and events was not psychosomatic. And with the discovery of the HIV virus, a theory could be put forward that explained these findings.

Of course, there are major differences between AIDS and CFIDS: (1) CFIDS is not fatal, and it tends to improve over time; (2) the HIV virus is not present in CFIDS; (3) the degree of immune deficiency is relatively mild in CFIDS; (4) the degree of fatigue is more severe in CFIDS; and (5) CFIDS is not spread by blood to blood contact. Despite these differences, the diseases have similarities.

*T*he Physician's Dilemma

CFIDS has brought medicine to a crossroads. Is this syndrome a vague collection of neurotic complaints, or a specific illness, radically different from any that medicine has trained itself to recognize?

The debate surrounding CFIDS among physicians has been difficult for patients and researchers alike. It is unlikely that physicians have ever before come across the particular set of circumstances encountered with this illness. While patients feel anger and frustration for the lack of involvement and knowledge by physicians on CFIDS, let us look at it from the doctor's perspective.

Modern medicine prides itself on scientific accuracy. The days of clinical medicine, listening to and trusting patients who may or may not be telling the truth, have been replaced with sophisticated machines and tests that do not lie. The art of medicine gave birth to an unruly child, medical technology. The old-fashioned doctor who listens carefully to the patient has become extinct, replaced by one more scientific and objective, one very conscious of potential legal problems. This new breed, pressed by economic realities, listens to the patient only long enough to decide which tests will give *the* scientific answer. Computerized cookbook medicine is the way of the future.

The malpractice crisis has speeded this change in the nature of medical practice. When a patient complains of numerous confusing symptoms, batteries of tests are ordered so that lawsuits may be avoided. Instead of carefully listening to and comforting patients, the physician focuses on self-protection. Physician and patient have ceased being allies and have become distrusting potential enemies.

Medical economics also contributes to the failure of modern medicine in the area of CFIDS. For a ten-minute surgical procedure an insurance company pays hundreds of dollars, whereas a one-hour visit reviewing the numerous symptoms of a complex illness is not covered at all. Results count, and surgical procedures render a result that can be seen on pathology reports. The one-hour discussion with a patient cannot be easily summarized. Patients' understanding, reassurance, comfort, and trust do not have a dollar value, and are thus not compensated.

There is an arrogance in modern medicine that seems to say there can be nothing new or undiscovered, except for a few details that only academicians are permitted to explore. The emphasis on the medical literature has closed the thinking minds of many physicians. We know it all, and are not interested in "new" observations. How could a disease like CFIDS have escaped our sophisticated study and perceptions all these years? If an illness is not clearly defined by the literature, it does not exist.

In many respects medical science is a primitive art. Volumes can be written about obscure and rare diseases with known enzyme defects, but general articles on poorly understood conditions are not acceptable because of the lack of hard, objective findings. Speculation is not acceptable. Prominent medical journals are reluctant to risk their reputations by publishing articles on a controversial illness. Suggestions that CFIDS might be related to yeast infections or food allergy are openly ridiculed. Researchers avoid the illness to avoid ridicule by their colleagues. Physicians must stick to medical doctrine or face censure.

Throughout history, physicians have been in the comfortable (or uncomfortable) position of "knowing" the art of healing. The science they studied was detailed and complicated, and completely out of reach of the patients who came to them for help. It took years of training and experience to understand the abnormal physiology that constituted disease. Physicians were used to saying, "We know and you do not." And usually they were right.

Even if they were wrong, patients never found out about it. They either died, or some complicated answer was invented to explain the apparent mistakes. Patients did not know the language of medicine, nor did they have any desire to learn.

But in the twentieth century this has changed. The public has become educated and sophisticated in learning those aspects of medicine that affect their lives. Every day the newspapers contain articles explaining everything from the mechanisms of arteriosclerosis to new surgical treatments for Alzheimer's disease. Patients join support groups, or read books like this one, thus gaining access to sophisticated medical information that may be unknown to the practicing physician. Parents of children with cystic fibrosis know far more about this disease than do the majority of physicians practicing in the United States today.

Although many physicians acknowledge that researching a disease may be helpful for patients, some are resentful when patients know more about a subject than they themselves do. It is extremely uncomfortable for a physician to be asked specific questions in an unfamiliar area by a patient who is supposed to be asking for help. The usual response to this is immediate referral to a specialist. Aside from admitting ignorance, it is the only way to handle the problem. And it is realistic. Patients so sophisticated that they know more than the physician need to be referred to someone else. Physicians have a choice: they can either admit their own ignorance or accuse patients of ignorance.

This, in part, has led to the uncomfortable position CFIDS patients face today. People ill with CFIDS have been unable to find help through conventional medical practices. They suffer with numerous symptoms and perceive that physicians do not take them seriously. Some of the more receptive physicians state that they do not yet know enough about this illness, but patients still hear them saying that they think it is not a real disease.

Physicians need to be cautious. In the long run, caution will more effectively sort through the issues involved in CFIDS research than will jumping to conclusions. Patience is necessary for real progress. But physicians should not deny the obvious and cite caution as an excuse. The evidence that CFIDS is an important medical condition is obvious, yet too many physicians and government health agencies do not recognize it and seem unwilling to open their minds.

For the researchers studying CFIDS, progress is painfully slow. For those suffering with it, patience is even more difficult to maintain. But it would be easier to tolerate the symptoms of CFIDS if patients could talk with and trust their physicians. The science of CFIDS is in its infancy, and until this science matures, physicians should not be afraid to listen to and support those who come to us for help. Physicians must discipline the unruly child, medical technology, and not abandon the art of medicine.

PART 2

Description of an Illness

CHAPTER 2

The Course of CFIDS

Now that we have a general idea of what CFIDS is, who gets it, and some of the controversy that surrounds it, we must take a closer look at the particular pattern of symptoms that is CFIDS.

The key to the diagnosis of CFIDS is an understanding of the underlying pattern of symptoms rather than an emphasis on the most prominent symptom. The physician must return to sound clinical medicine, taking a complete medical history and listening to the entire range of symptoms in order to observe the underlying pattern. This is a throwback to the grand old days of clinical medicine when the symptoms of an illness were studied in detail. The mark of modern medicine is to jump to the lab test that will give the answer in the least amount of time. We practice "game show medicine": the patient begins to relate symptoms, and the first doctor to ring the buzzer with the correct answer wins. This approach simply does not work with the CFIDS patient.

For example, I know one woman who had severe headaches that began after an apparent viral illness. She did not feel well generally and communicated this to her physician, but the doctor's concern was with the headaches. She had a full headache evaluation, including an electroencephalogram (EEG) and computerized X ray (CT scan) of the brain, all of which were negative. She was then sent to a neurologist, who noted her memory and concentration problems, light-headedness, and numbness of her hands and feet while lying still. Brain tumor, multiple sclerosis, and a host of other serious neurological diseases were considered. When tests for those conditions proved negative, an inappropriate diagnosis of depression was made.

However, from the onset of this woman's illness the pattern of her symptoms was typical for CFIDS, and had they been explored, the patient might have been spared considerable expense and distress. Neither her original physician nor her neurologist ever asked her about the flulike malaise, sore throats, abdominal discomfort, joint and muscle pain, lymph node tenderness, and eye pain. After six months without a diagnosis, the fatigue and malaise displaced headaches as the most disabling symptom. At that time the diagnosis of CFIDS was considered.

Sometimes, inadvertently, a patient can add to the difficulties of diagnosis. During an initial evaluation, patients with CFIDS describe in great detail their exhaustion and fatigue. They can eloquently verbalize the effect of this symptom on their activity and how it aggravates all the other symptoms. It is the usual cause of their disability. But, at the end of an interview, when I ask a patient to list the three most severe and disabling symptoms, fatigue often is not mentioned. They list headaches, joint pain, muscle aches, memory loss, and other symptoms. When I ask about the exhaustion, they frequently say, "Oh yes, fatigue really is the worst symptom, I forgot about that." The fatigue is so pervasive and constant that it is overlooked in listing symptoms. Fatigue is the key to the overall pattern of discomfort. It lies immediately behind and pervades all other symptoms, and must be explored by the physician.

The Diagnosis

The diagnostic criteria published by the Centers for Disease Control in 1988 provides guidelines for the diagnosis of CFIDS involving both major or absolute criteria necessary for the diagnosis and minor or variable criteria. These criteria may be summarized as follows (Holmes 88):

Major Criteria:

1. New onset of severe fatigue for six months or more, causing at least a 50 percent activity reduction
2. Exclusion of other illnesses causing similar symptoms

Minor Criteria (eight or more):

  Symptom Criteria

  1. Mild fever
  2. Sore throat
  3. Painful or swollen lymph nodes
  4. Generalized muscle weakness
  5. Muscle discomfort
  6. Fatigue worsened by exercise
  7. Headaches
  8. Neuropsychologic complaints
  9. Sleep disturbance
  10. Acute onset of symptom complex

Physical Examination Criteria (two of three):

  1. Fever
  2. Throat inflammation
  3. Palpable or tender lymph nodes

It should be noted that these criteria were designed for research purposes, and as such were meant to be restrictive. Moreover, these criteria are not appropriate for children, as will be discussed later.

It is theoretically possible that some people may have this illness in a mild form that can be dismissed as normal stresses and strains, occasional headaches, abdominal discomfort, and fatigue. There is no simple and obvious marker to show where "normal" ends and "disease" begins. But although CFIDS patients have symptoms that are similar to the normal complaints of daily life, in CFIDS they are severe and debilitating. They cause a marked reduction of daily activity that significantly limits a person. This activity reduction and disability defines the illness more than any individual symptom.

In discussing the clinical presentation and symptom pattern of CFIDS I refer to patients with severe symptoms, not the minor fatigue and somatic symptoms that everyone has. Perhaps this is arbitrary, and it may be that twenty years from now this separation will prove false. But for our present purposes CFIDS is a severe illness that causes a significant limitation of daily activities over prolonged periods of time.

Onset—The Turbulent First Six Months

For up to a third of patients who are eventually diagnosed with CFIDS, the first six months are a period of indescribable turbulence. The sudden disruption of good health, the confusion, the multitude of doctor visits, the tests and procedures, the changing or fluctuating symptoms, the fear and expense, the problems with work or school—all conspire to create a nightmare that compounds the problem of being ill. More than one patient has said they wished they could be diagnosed with terminal cancer just so they would know what was happening to them.

For another 25 percent the onset is gradual or insidious, sometimes so slow that they do not recognize any illness. They experience a mild fatigue, some depression, occasional migraines. The illness is recognized only months later when the entire symptom complex evolves to a disabling degree. There is no initial turbulence for these patients because of the gentle and gradual onset.

Some patients have an acute onset of symptoms, but aside from the difficulty in establishing a diagnosis, there is little turbulence. An acute flulike illness and symptoms of daily fatigue, headaches, muscle aches, and joint pain persist. The patients can tolerate the symptoms, but not the changing explanations of physicians. The symptoms fluctuate little and the overall clinical course is relatively constant.

Because of the difficulty in establishing a diagnosis, there is no firm agreement among researchers as to the percentage of patients who have a severe, complicated onset of symptoms. Patients with turbulent onset patterns usually have one or two symptoms that are dominant and attract diagnostic attention. The diagnosis of CFIDS is not made until later when the entire symptom pattern becomes apparent. At that time the original dominant symptom fades in importance and other symptoms of the pattern dominate. Because the diagnosis of CFIDS rests on the entire symptom pattern, early diagnosis can be difficult. However, if the physician has the symptom pattern of CFIDS in mind, the period of confusion can be shortened. The purpose of this section is to discuss the period of the first six months, particularly in patients who are very ill.

*A*cute Onset?

It is often said that up to 75 percent of patients with CFIDS have an acute onset of illness. But on close questioning, many, perhaps the majority, had mild symptoms suggestive of the illness prior to the acute onset. Do patients have an acute onset of CFIDS or is preexisting CFIDS acutely worsened? Did the illness actually begin with the acute episode? The difficulty in answering this question is that the symptoms of CFIDS are nonspecific, and nearly everyone has them to a mild degree. It is possible that patients merely recall normal nonspecific symptoms once they develop severe CFIDS.

I have evaluated several professional athletes, and their interesting observations represent a clue to this bizarre illness. Many athletes are excellent observers of themselves and their physical abilities—a quality few of us have. As such, their testimony is extremely useful. One, a swimmer, was in perfect physical health. He was young, well disciplined, and of near Olympic caliber. He swam daily and was finely tuned to any changes in stamina and health. He developed typical CFIDS, and on first questioning he had a typical acute onset—one day he developed the "flu" and did not recover for the next three years. However, closer questioning revealed some interesting details.

He had noticed that for about three weeks prior to the onset of his illness, his legs would ache after his daily laps. His overall strength was unchanged, but his performance was slightly impaired with decreased sprint times. As a disciplined athlete he noticed this change because there was no reasonable explanation for it. There was an isolated aching in his legs that he had never experienced before. He dismissed these aches as trivial; he was otherwise well. Yet when he developed CFIDS these symptoms became a prominent part of his illness: muscle aching, weakness, and a rubbery sensation in his legs.

Another athlete had similar observations. This man, a runner in his late thirties, ran in a disciplined manner for many years. He had run marathons in his youth but now limited himself to seven or eight miles daily. He observed a slight change in his performance ability for several weeks before becoming ill. Specifically, he noticed that at around the fifth or sixth mile he became tired, a phenomenon that was unusual for him. (Actually, when I heard him explain this I had to suppress a smile; if I ever reached mile five on a run I would be ready for autopsy.)

He paid little attention to this observation and continued his running without interruption. About three weeks later his two-year-old son developed a fever. His wife also developed a fever and what appeared to be the flu. Two days later he also developed the flu: fever, aching, sore throat, lymph node tenderness. Typical, ordinary flu. His wife and child responded normally with recovery in about a week, but the man has not recovered. He persisted with symptoms since the day he developed the flu and has had a course typical of CFIDS.

This man's case is interesting in several respects. He is an intelligent, well-adjusted, motivated professional with no sign of emotional illness in his evaluation. The implication of CFIDS being a psychosomatic illness is unjustified in his case. Also although he would be considered to have an acute onset of symptoms, he could date the real onset of his illness to a subtle change three weeks earlier. It was almost trivial in nature, yet appears to be related to the subsequent development of CFIDS. The symptom during this three-week period, the fatigue at mile five or six, marked the "vulnerable period" of CFIDS in this man. It appears that this athlete's illness was triggered by an apparently benign viral infection that caused no difficulties for his wife and child.

The existence of a vulnerable state is not proven, and is nearly impossible to test because of the mild, commonplace nature of the symptoms. Perhaps it represents an increased vigilance to the trivial symptoms of everyday life. Perhaps it is a genuine phenomenon indicating that the true cause of CFIDS may enter silently, like a stealth bomber.

Concept of Trigger Event

The variety of trigger events can be bewildering, contributing to the confusion in the turbulent first six months. In this discussion we will be considering patients with acute onset of symptoms, keeping in mind that many had prior hints of a change in their health.

Perhaps the most frequent trigger event is an acute viral infection. It is not clear whether certain viruses are more likely than others to be a trigger for CFIDS, but if so, viruses such as Epstein-Barr and Coxsackie would be likely candidates. Nonviral events also can mark the beginning of CFIDS. Exposure to certain chemicals, bacterial infections, emotional stress, surgical procedures, physical injury, immunizations, and physical stress have all been trigger events in patients I have evaluated.

One patient was well until an automobile accident, after which she developed the range and pattern of symptoms of CFIDS. Batteries of tests were done to evaluate these symptoms, felt to be due to the automobile accident. The tests, of course, were normal and showed no tissue injury. The insurance company believed her to be malingering for financial gain in a future lawsuit.

Another patient had the acute onset of symptoms while working with certain chemicals at his place of employment. He was bedridden for several months with the possible diagnosis of toxic encephalopathy from exposure to industrial solvents. But the tests came back negative, and being away from the chemicals did not improve his symptoms. Again the company assumed malingering, while the patient believed the company was covering up toxic chemical exposure.

Another patient developed infectious mononucleosis and did not recover for months.

The list is nearly endless, and the nature of the precipitating event adds to the confusion. But does it really make a difference?

If the man in the last example had not developed infectious mononucleosis, would he have had an acute onset a week later with some other event? This issue remains unresolved and controversial among researchers. Is CFIDS a specific disease that can be triggered by many different events, or is it a collection of separate diseases? We will examine this question in greater detail in a future chapter.

Clinical Course

The typical course is characterized by the persistence of the symptoms on a constant basis for a prolonged period of time. Although the diagnosis is not made until the symptoms persist for at least six months, patients who are ill at three months with a typical pattern of symptoms are still ill at six months. It is quite likely, therefore, that a three-month history of typical symptoms after acute onset is sufficient for the diagnosis. How many people may contract CFIDS and have a spontaneous resolution of symptoms within six months is not known. This information should become available over the next few years.

Different individuals may have specific symptoms that cause the greatest problems, but over half of patients say that fatigue is the worst. The remainder complain that headaches, muscle pain, joint pain, abdominal pain, or lymphatic pain is the worst symptom. Except for dizziness, the neurologic symptoms frequently do not become prominent until some months after the acute presentation.

Another hallmark of this illness is the presence of relapses and remissions, although some patients, perhaps 30 percent, have a steady course without dramatic fluctuations. The relapses, or periods of marked worsening of symptoms, may follow a variety of factors, including viral or bacterial infections, allergic exposure, stress, hormone changes, or exercise. In some patients the relapses have no clear antecedent causes. Some patients state that relapses occur just when symptoms are beginning to improve. It has been my experience that the months of November and March seem to be particularly difficult for patients with CFIDS, perhaps because of the prevalence of viral infections.

*S*ymptoms

The beginning of this chapter listed the diagnostic criteria published by the Centers for Disease Control. A more detailed account of these symptoms follows.

Fatigue

The vast majority of patients state that although they occasionally have relatively good periods, they never have days when their level of energy or exercise tolerance is as good as on an average day before they became ill. The fatigue is not merely tiredness, as can be experienced by anyone after exertion, but is described as exhaustion or malaise. It may come on suddenly, and some people have described going out for a walk and experiencing a sudden onset of exhaustion so severe that they were afraid they would not be able to return home. Waves of fatigue, often accompanied by nausea, frequently follow minor activities such as housecleaning or yard work. Many patients describe this exhaustion as the primary underlying symptom of the syndrome, and that all other symptoms, such as headache, abdominal discomfort, and joint pain, fluctuate with the fatigue.

Neurologic and Neuropsychiatric Symptoms

Numerous symptoms fall into this category, and 97 percent of CFIDS patients experience at least some of them. The most common are short-term memory loss and inability to concentrate. Patients may get lost driving on familiar roads near their house or be unable to understand simple paragraphs in books or newspapers. It may be difficult to recall familiar words or names. These symptoms tend to be the most common reason that people are unable to work.

Other neurologic symptoms include abnormal sensations (paresthesias) such as numbness or tingling, and occasional episodes of burning in the hands and feet. Dizziness is common and is often present during the acute onset. Light-headedness, fainting spells, muscle twitching, balance problems, abnormal movements, and seizures also occur. Although not strictly a neurologic symptom, sleep disturbance is present in almost all patients, consisting of either hypersomnolence, insomnia, or both. An almost constant symptom is the inability to feel refreshed after sleep. Due to the extent and importance of these symptoms, they will be discussed in greater detail later.

Neuropsychiatric complaints are present in at least 60 percent of patients and can be characterized by changes in emotions as compared to their state prior to becoming ill. Depression and anxiety or panic attacks occur frequently. Among the most devastating of all symptoms are emotional changes in combination with fatigue and neurologic symptoms that create an inability to cope. This is particularly aggravated when medical consultation fails to recognize that the symptoms have an organic cause.

Headache

The headaches of CFIDS are of two kinds. The most common is pain in the frontal region surrounding the sinuses or in the forehead. A second type of headache, and frequently distinct from these frontal headaches, is a pressure sensation in the base of the skull, and this tends to be more severe. The headaches can be confused with typical migraine, and for 20 percent of patients with CFIDS they are the most severe symptom. "Brain ache" is a term some patients use for the discomfort and worsening of headaches that may follow attempts to read or concentrate.

Abdominal Pain

Numerous abdominal symptoms are associated with CFIDS, and most patients are diagnosed as having irritable bowel syndrome. Pain in the abdomen may be prominent, and is localized either in the midabdomen, or in the liver and spleen areas. Most patients complain of gas, bloating, distention, and periods of diarrhea and/or constipation. Vomiting occasionally occurs and is associated with particularly severe abdominal symptoms.

Sore Throat

Only rarely is the sore throat severe. It is usually described as a scratchy feeling, and may be present daily, especially in the morning. Smokers usually dismiss the sore throat as being due to cigarettes. Some patients have periods of sore throat that last for several days at a time and are more painful. Mouth ulcers are common, and thrush, or oral candidiasis, is occasionally present.

Lymphatic Pain

This symptom is present in 70 percent of CFIDS patients. The lymph nodes are tender in multiple areas, such as in the front and back of the neck, armpits, elbows, and groin. Patients notice swelling of the lymph nodes, but only rarely does this swelling impress their physicians. The patient will feel a lymph node because of its tenderness and become aware of subtle changes in size, but the swelling does not become abnormal from the physician's point of view. Any truly large lymph node should be biopsied because this is uncommon in CFIDS. One of the most characteristic symptoms is pain in the subauricular lymph nodes, the nodes located under the ear and behind the angle of the jaw. This pain typically accompanies symptoms of dizziness, hearing changes, or ear pain.

Joint Pain

Pain in the joints is present in about 70 percent of patients and is usually not severe. The most common joints affected are the knees, ankles, elbows, and hips, but pain in the fingers also occurs. Very rarely is there redness, heat, or swelling of the joints.

Muscle Pain

Aching in the muscles is common, and many patients have it on a constant basis. It is described as a flulike aching that exercise makes worse. It may also present as sharp pain in specific muscle groups, and many patients with prominent muscle pain are diagnosed as having fibrositis or fibromyalgia. Prominent also is the sensation of muscle weakness. On occasion, there is atrophy of specific muscle groups, a shrinking in size, that may be obvious to the patient. However, although the muscles may feel weak to the patient, muscle strength testing is usually normal. This paradox has generated a lively debate among researchers and will be discussed more fully in a later chapter.

Eye Pain/Light Sensitivity

Patients often complain of aching behind their eyes, frequently along the upper ridge of the orbit. Light hurts their eyes, a condition known as photophobia, which is particularly distressing during night driving when the glare of headlights can be uncomfortable. Scratchy, dry eyes and disturbances of vision with blurring are also common. Detailed examination by ophthalmologists usually reveals them to be normal, however, with the possible exception of the Schirmer test, which measures tear production.

Fever/Chills/Night Sweats

Patients with CFIDS almost always have abnormal temperature sensations. Actually, true fever is relatively rare after the first few months of illness, but patients feel as if they have a fever. If the temperature is measured at these times, it is often below normal. Most patients do not tolerate cold temperatures well; a few feel worse with heat. Night sweats are less common, but may be dramatic, particularly in the first year of the illness.

Rash

Two types of rash are seen in CFIDS. The most common, a flushing of the cheeks, is present in about 60 percent of patients.

The flushing can appear suddenly and at unpredictable times. For some, the flushing regularly follows minor exertion. However, this flushing is minor and usually unnoticed. Indeed, the "rosy cheek" appearance may be interpreted as a sign of good health. It may be the first symptom in patients with a gradual onset of symptoms, and some patients describe a mild itching when the flush is present. About 20 percent have a second rash, a fine, lacelike rash on the neck and chest that may persist independently of the flushing. Many patients with this type of rash have it daily.

Palpitations

Perhaps up to 40 percent of patients with CFIDS have palpitations and/or chest pain that is particularly disturbing. A fluttering sensation in the midchest, accompanied by an irregular heartbeat, can be frightening. Usually, patients are told that the palpitations are the normal fluttering that occurs with stress, anxiety, and too much caffeine. It is rare that significant or dangerous heart disease is found. In many patients the palpitations are due to mitral valve prolapse, an extremely common condition in which the mitral valve of the heart is floppy.

Palpitations are a good example of a "normal" symptom that is abnormal because of its pattern in CFIDS. The palpitations are probably not due to tissue damage in the heart, and are instead set off by the same mechanism that is present in regular anxiety. But there is frequently no clear relationship between the palpitations and anxiety in patients with CFIDS.

Shortness of Breath

Patients may complain of episodes of shortness of breath, not associated with wheezing, coughing, or airway obstruction. The sensation frequently passes in less than a minute, but it causes patients to take deep breaths, as if they are experiencing "air hunger."

Allergies

Up to 60 percent of CFIDS patients have allergies. Many never had allergies before; some notice a marked worsening of previously mild allergies. Marked sensitivities occur to drugs and chemical odors. As many as 30 percent of patients with CFIDS had a history of asthma prior to becoming ill. A history of allergies and/or asthma has been noted in several studies on CFIDS and may represent a genetic marker that identifies a group of people who are at risk for the illness.

Weight Changes

Many patients notice unusual fluctuations of their weight. The most common pattern is weight loss at the onset of the illness, followed by weight gain. These changes do not clearly correlate with changes in food consumption. The weight gain way be aggravated by inactivity caused by fatigue.

Physical Examination

An essential part of the physician's evaluation in any disease state is to observe changes in the size, shape, or appearance of the body's organs. In CFIDS, the physical examination is remarkably consistent from patient to patient. It forms a pattern that changes little over time except for fluctuations in severity.

One common misunderstanding is that the physical examination in CFIDS is "normal." Abnormalities are almost always present, but they are subtle. A patient with CFIDS looks quite healthy. He or she may be housebound or even bedridden but, when sitting on the examining table in the doctor's office, looks well. In CFIDS, unlike most other illnesses, there is usually no objective evidence of damage to the body tissues—whatever is causing the symptoms is doing so through a mechanism that is not causing obvious harm. The abnormalities seen on physical examination in CFIDS are due to pain and tenderness of tissues, but without obvious injury.

The physician needs to perform the physical examination with an eye to what is expected and what is unusual, first carefully scrutinizing for evidence of another pathological process, such as hepatitis, malignancy, or thyroid disease. Severe abnormalities, such as a goiter, a large liver, or a dramatic heart murmur, are usually not seen, and if present they imply either a coexisting condition or another diagnosis. The physician also should watch for a pattern of "soft" abnormalities consistent with what is expected in CFIDS.

The following discussion is somewhat technical and may be difficult for nonmedical readers. But the examination described is an ordinary one that any physician can perform, and it may be helpful for patients to understand what their doctor is looking for.

Skin

The skin may show several changes. There may be pallor, resembling anemia. This pallor is sometimes interrupted by a flushing rash on the cheeks, extending down onto the neck. Another type of rash that may be present is a fine, lacelike one on the neck and chest; it is usually constant and does not come and go like the flushing. There may be itching of the skin and, rarely, hives. Dermatographism is often present, a prominent red line on the skin after stroking.

Patients with CFIDS state that they bruise easily, but generalized bruising is rarely seen. There may be thinning of the hair, and interestingly, the fingerpads may be atrophic so that the fingerprints are difficult to see. The skin may be red and shiny, changes that usually occur after the illness has been present for a substantial period of time. In two patients I have seen striae, purple skin lines associated with a variety of rheumatic conditions.

Eyes

The most prominent abnormality on examination of the eyes is photophobia, discomfort with bright light. The eye structures are usually normal, as are the muscle movements and vision on general screening, but light sensitivity is noted during the examination. The moisture production of the eyes is often decreased, and because of this finding some patients are told they have a condition known as Sjogren's syndrome. However, the specific antibody tests for Sjogren's syndrome are usually normal. Mild inflammation of the whites of the eyes is sometimes seen. Patients with double vision, atrophy of the optic nerve, or inflammation inside the eye need specialized examinations and usually have another illness, since these conditions are rarely seen in CFIDS.

Ears

Although many CFIDS patients have ringing and pain in their ears, the examination of the ear canals and eardrums is almost always normal. One interesting and almost invariable finding is that in those patients who complain of earache, tenderness in the lymph node just under the ear, the subauricular lymph node, is found.

Throat

The most common of the numerous signs in the mouth is redness of the throat, or pharyngitis, especially when the patient is experiencing pain in the throat. Pus on the pharynx or tonsils is unusual, however. Many times a patient has a very sore throat but the pharynx looks relatively normal. Mouth ulcers occur frequently. Ten to twenty percent of patients with severe CFIDS will have signs of thrush, an oral yeast infection, in the mouth. This appears as a white coating of the tongue or cheeks that does not easily scrape off. When this occurs, a culture for candida may confirm thrush, and specialized tests may be appropriate.

Neck

Examination of the neck and attention to the thyroid is very important. It is not uncommon for the thyroid to be somewhat tender, and if so, thyroid antibodies should be obtained. The thyroid should be of normal size and shape without nodules or masses.

Lymph Nodes

Examination of the lymph nodes is, for me, the key to the physical examination. The hallmark of this examination is that the nodes are of normal size but are tender. A second related unusual characteristic is that patients know the location of the lymph nodes because of the pain they experience. That a patient can accurately localize the epitrochlear, scalene, or subauricular lymph nodes is striking. Patients with CFIDS frequently point to these locations without knowing that lymph nodes are there. Only about 60 percent of CFIDS patients have tender lymph nodes. If there is significant, persistent swelling in one or several nodes, serious consideration should be given to lymph node biopsy.

Chest

Physical examination of the chest is usually normal.

Heart

The heart is usually normal without evidence of enlargement or inflammation. The heart rate is often mildly elevated, up to 110 beats per minute. A murmur due to mitral valve prolapse may be heard. It is not known whether this is more common in CFIDS or if it is just diagnosed more commonly to explain the palpitations.

Abdomen

Abnormalities found on palpation of the abdomen are also very common and, as with the lymph nodes, consist of tenderness without organ enlargement. Tenderness in the liver and spleen areas, under the rib cage margins on the right and left sides, is seen. Generalized tenderness in the midabdomen without swelling or masses may also be seen. Organ enlargement or masses are not a part of CFIDS and require further investigation. Tenderness in the groin is frequently due to pain in the lymph nodes of this area.

Genitalia

Tenderness is sometimes noted without signs of enlargement, masses, or specific infections.

Muscles

Muscle tenderness is common and is frequently accompanied by specific trigger points. These points are small areas of increased tenderness within the bulk of the muscles, to the degree that the patient may wince when the area is palpated. Testing of strength and tone is usually normal, except in severely ill patients who have muscle atrophy.

Neurological

On superficial examination there are usually no abnormalities. However, on careful examination, anywhere from 10 to 20 percent of patients have minor abnormalities, the most common of which is poor balance, particularly with the eyes closed. Lower extremity tendon reflexes may be increased. In general, the cranial nerves, mental status, and cognitive function are normal on routine exam. Detailed cognitive testing, however, may reveal abnormalities.

In summary, in CFIDS cases nearly everything—the lymph nodes, muscles, liver, and spleen—is tender to palpation, yet these organs are of normal size, shape, and consistency. If any swelling or other variation is noted, specific diagnostic workup should be directed by the physician to look for other possible causes of the symptoms.

The Neurology of CFIDS

Along with exhaustion, the symptoms arising from the nervous system are the most disabling for patients with CFIDS. The neurologic symptoms themselves form an unusual pattern, although not specific to this syndrome. Most informal studies have shown that they are experienced by nearly all CFIDS patients. Because of the frequency of neurologic symptoms and their importance in causing disability, this section will explore them in greater detail.

CFIDS patients have symptoms that appear to involve the brain, spinal cord, and peripheral nerves. The most common symptom is headache, followed by dizziness and difficulty with concentration and memory (cognitive disturbances). For some patients, particularly children, these symptoms are mild and merely annoying, and do not compete with the more severe symptoms of fatigue and malaise. The degree of neurologic symptoms in this group seems to parallel the degree of fatigue. But the presence of these symptoms is so standard in CFIDS that I would be very reluctant to make the diagnosis without them.

For some patients, perhaps 20 percent, the neurologic symptoms are severe and cause more disability than all other symptoms combined. These patients are referred to neurologists for evaluation and multiple diagnostic procedures. The greatest concern for this subgroup of patients is multiple sclerosis, and differentiation of the two illnesses may be very difficult.

Neurologists have been reluctant to recognize the pattern of neurologic symptoms because of their relatively nonspecific nature, minor physical examination abnormalities, and normal standard laboratory evaluations. Prior to recognizing the illness, I referred my first adult CFIDS patients to a variety of neurologists. I was worried that these adults had multiple sclerosis, not only because of their symptoms but because Upstate New York is part of the "MS belt." The neurologists stated that none of the patients had MS, which I accepted as true, but the diagnoses ranged from Huntington's chorea to depression. A single patient who saw three different neurologists emerged with three different diagnoses, and this variety implied that all were wrong.

The degree and progression of the neurologic symptoms are perhaps the most sensitive hints to the prognosis for CFIDS patients. If a patient has an acute onset of symptoms and subsequently develops only minor neurologic symptoms, I am most optimistic about resolution of the illness over the next few years. The first sign of resolution is usually improvement of the neurologic symptoms. However, if a patient has severe neurologic symptoms at the onset, or if there is steady worsening of these symptoms over the first two or three years, the chances of recovery plummet, even if the mononucleosis-like symptoms (sore throat, joint pain, fevers, sweats, lymph node pain) improve.

An overview of the central nervous system symptoms of CFIDS was discussed previously, but because of the importance of these symptoms, let us examine them in greater detail. In a study done in 1986 on one hundred patients with CFIDS, using a standardized questionnaire, over 95 percent of patients had neurologic symptoms, not including recurrent headache.

Memory loss	88%
Difficulty with concentration	82%
Dizziness	76%
Paresthesias	63%
Muscle twitching	62%
Word-finding difficulty	60%
Ringing in ears	49%
Balance disturbance	36%
Fainting spells	26%
Involuntary movements	24%
Seizures	6%

Memory Loss

Nearly all CFIDS patients observe difficulty with memory, particularly short-term memory. It is common to hear of patients unable to remember phone numbers, friends' names, even the address of their house. Patients develop habits to circumvent this symptom such as carrying a note pad, or leaving clues around the house to remind themselves of ordinary daily matters such as turning off the stove. Some patients are disabled by this cognitive symptom, particularly those in jobs requiring strong cognitive skills.

Difficulty with Concentration, Word Finding

CFIDS patients have difficulty in focusing and maintaining attention. It is common to hear patients describe the inability to follow simple paragraphs while reading or understand the plot of television programs. Some investigators have related both the inability to concentrate and loss of short-term memory to the general symptom of fatigue, whereas others have maintained that these represent specific neurological deficits. An ongoing controversy exists about the presence of dementia, a severe loss of cognitive skills. I have no doubt that dementia exists in some patients, but not in patients with the usual degree of severity. Other cognitive abnormalities may be present, although they are less often noted by patients. Word-finding difficulty may be present, as are difficulties with spatial orientation.

Dizziness, Fainting Spells, Ringing in Ears

These symptoms, also common, may be the most frequent reason why patients with CFIDS go to the emergency room. The dizziness is distressing and associated with anxiety, panic attacks, and unusual somatic sensations. In the emergency room, however, physicians diagnose either acute anxiety reaction or labrinthitis, a disturbance of the middle ear. These diagnoses would be appropriate were it not for the rest of the symptoms of CFIDS, which are rarely explored.

Dizziness or light-headedness is most pronounced on changing positions. Fainting spells may occur, but only rarely does a patient completely lose consciousness. It is even more rare for patients to lose consciousness without warning, so automobile accidents and falls down a stairway are uncommon. However, a patient who has these spells should not drive.

Paresthesias

Paresthesias are abnormal sensations, such as numbness, shooting pains, and burning, in the peripheral nerves. The most common of these in CFIDS is numbness in the hands and feet, particularly while lying still or going to sleep. With motion of the extremities, the numbness may disappear. Some patients are troubled by shooting pains or "electrical shocks" in the extremities. Pain in the upper spinal cord or base of the spine may occur. Some patients have burning sensations in the fingers to the degree that they are unable to hold a pencil. Muscle twitching is usually little more than an annoying symptom. It is of interest, however, that although many symptoms exist implying disease of the peripheral nerves, specific testing of these nerves with standard electromyography (EMG) and nerve conduction velocity studies is almost always normal.

Urinary Frequency

Specific questioning concerning urinary symptoms is very important. A small minority of patients will have incontinence (inability to control the urine), but this symptom in CFIDS is intermittent and not progressive. If incontinence is severe or progressive, a diagnosis of multiple sclerosis is strongly suggested.

Although incontinence is unusual, urinary frequency and pain on urination are not. The most common explanation given to patients with these symptoms is recurrent urinary tract infection, but no bacteria are isolated from the urine. Occasionally the frequency and pain are so intense that the diagnosis of interstitial cystitis is made. This subject is mentioned in this section only because it is possible that abnormalities in the autonomic nervous system account for these symptoms.

Balance Disturbance, Involuntary Movements, Seizures

Some patients with CFIDS have more dramatic neurologic abnormalities, but fortunately these are rare. It is in this group of patients that differentiation from MS and other neurologic diseases is difficult. In my experience, up to 10 percent of children have some form of seizure disorder in addition to the symptoms of CFIDS.

Fatigue and Pain as Neurologic Symptoms

Fatigue

The origin of the fatigue seen in CFIDS is a subject of ongoing debate among researchers. It is extraordinary that we know so little about the causes of fatigue, a common phenomenon. The debate involves whether the fatigue of CFIDS originates in the brain (central fatigue) or in the rest of the body (peripheral fatigue). An example of the latter type would be disease in the muscles or mitochondria, the energy processing units of cells. The debate has been particularly heated across the Atlantic. Researchers in Great Britain have supported the muscle/mitochondria theory, whereas many in the United States feel that the fatigue is central.

Patients complain of extreme fatigue and exhaustion. They also relate muscle weakness as a specific symptom, yet testing of specific muscle strength is usually normal. Minor abnormalities may be found, but the weakness described by the patient is so dramatic that it cannot be explained by these minor abnormalities.

That fatigue can be caused by disease in the brain has been known for years. It is an extremely complex area of neurology, involving parts of the brain that are difficult to test by methods available to us. However, in general, diseases involving the frontal lobes and the midbrain will cause fatigue, and I feel that central fatigue is a plausible explanation for the symptom.

Pain

Pain is another hallmark of CFIDS. Pain is present in the abdomen, muscles, and joints; patients have headaches, lymph node pain, and sore throat. Physicians skeptical of CFIDS have said, "Everything hurts, but nothing is wrong." But pain in different organs in patients with CFIDS may not be due to disease in these organs. The primary abnormality may be an alteration in the perception of pain because of central nervous system disease. The pain of CFIDS may be another central symptom, reflecting disease in the brain rather than in the rest of the body.

An interesting phenomenon is the occurrence of pain at a site of previous injury. For example, a patient may have broken an ankle ten years prior to becoming ill with CFIDS, and it healed normally causing no discomfort. It is common to hear that with the onset of CFIDS, pain at the site of the old fracture returns. Surgical scars begin to hurt after a patient develops CFIDS, and minor injuries may cause severe pain. In one study, I examined ten patients by skin biopsy. The skin biopsies, a trivial procedure, were normal, but I was amazed at the degree of discomfort the biopsies caused, pain that sometimes lasted for months. In each of these instances it is clear that the degree of injury does not justify the amount of pain. Some physicians call this hypochondriasis, but it may be due to an abnormality within the brain, the part that regulates perception of pain.

The perception of pain is regulated in part by a portion of the nervous system called the autonomic nervous system. This region of the nervous system controls functions that are handled automatically, such as breathing, temperature regulation, and sweating. In CFIDS patients, there are numerous minor symptoms that may relate to a disturbance in autonomic function, such as abnormal temperature sensations, flushing of the cheeks, abnormal sweating, hives on the skin after scratching, and altered pain perception. Dizzy spells and light-headedness may be related to blood pressure variations, again indirectly due to autonomic disturbance. Rapid heart beat, palpitations, and periods of breathlessness also may be explained by autonomic nervous system dysfunction.

It is in this area that mind and body are hard to separate. For example, the autonomic nervous system prepares the body for emergencies with the "fight or flight" response. If a person, while strolling in the woods, came face to face with a grizzly bear, the autonomic nervous system would cause certain reactions in the body. Resources would become mobilized with rapid heart beat, and adrenal hormones would be pushed into the bloodstream to allow the person to respond appropriately to the crisis at hand. What is experienced is a panic attack, quite reasonable under the circumstances. Patients with CFIDS commonly have panic attacks but without external cause. It has been hypothesized that these panic attacks are another indication of autonomic nervous system abnormalities.

Abnormalities in the autonomic nervous system are seen in many illnesses affecting the brain. Skin studies in fibromyalgia, possibly the same illness as CFIDS, have shown changes indicating autonomic dysfunction. In CFIDS, preliminary studies have been able to document some of these abnormalities, but more detailed studies are needed.

Most patients and physicians have the impression that CFIDS is a form of chronic mononucleosis, affecting numerous areas of the body yet sparing the nervous system. However, many of the symptoms, including exhaustion, may actually result from a disease process affecting the brain. This one question, whether the symptoms of CFIDS are central or peripheral, is perhaps the most pressing issue requiring resolution, particularly important in developing treatment strategies.

That so few papers have been published concerning the abnormal neurologic testing seen in patients with CFIDS is unfortunate. However, a consensus among researchers has developed that there are specific laboratory abnormalities that, although not diagnostic in themselves, may be of value. Preliminary studies documenting abnormalities seen in magnetic resonance imaging (MRI), beam scan (a computerized EEG), SPECT scan (a study of brain blood flow), and cognitive function testing have been presented at several recent scientific conferences by numerous researchers. It is hoped that these papers will soon be published, allowing physicians access to technical information that will help to clarify difficult diagnostic problems.

Conclusion

CFIDS is a tremendously complex illness with myriad symptoms that partially resemble many other diseases. But the process of sorting through the symptoms and carefully looking for abnormalities on physical examination is no different from that of other illnesses. Like other illnesses, the symptoms of CFIDS form a specific pattern that, combined with the characteristic physical examination, is diagnostic. The difficulty in establishing a diagnosis of CFIDS should be resolved in the next few years as physicians become more familiar with this difficult and frustrating illness.

CHAPTER 3

Could It Be Something Else?

As we've seen, it is possible to diagnose CFIDS given at least moderate activity limitation and a typical pattern of symptoms. Why, then, has there been so much difficulty in making the diagnosis? Because CFIDS can be confused with other illnesses, anxiety, and depression.

Multiple Sclerosis

One of the greatest diagnostic problems for CFIDS patients with severe neurologic symptoms is to rule out MS as the cause. Multiple sclerosis is a disease that shares many features with CFIDS, including fatigue and neurologic symptoms. In most patients, however, differences in the pattern of symptoms allow differentiation of the two illnesses. MS patients rarely have muscle pain, lymph node pain, rash, or sore throat. MS patients usually feel worse in hot weather, whereas most CFIDS patients improve with heat.

The cause of MS is the presence of sclerotic plaques, which can be thought of as scar tissue within the brain. The majority of patients with MS have steady worsening and progression of their illness, but some have symptoms that remit. Like all diseases, multiple sclerosis has specific criteria that need to be met before a diagnosis can be made. Patients with CFIDS do not fit these criteria, but because they are close in symptoms, the diagnosis of atypical MS may be applied, one more name on the growing list. If a patient meets the diagnostic criteria for multiple sclerosis, known by all neurologists, then the diagnosis would be MS and not CFIDS. The treatments should conform to current remedies known to be of benefit in MS.

In the patients I have evaluated, nearly 5 percent have neurologic symptoms severe enough to be considered atypical MS. None fits the criteria of multiple sclerosis, and all have the full symptom complex of CFIDS. However, none of these patients has evolved into multiple sclerosis, even though they have now been followed for up to five years. It is a contradiction that needs to be addressed in future studies.

*D*epression

Perhaps the most bitter argument surrounding chronic fatigue / immune dysfunction syndrome concerns the role played by depression. Since the first descriptions of the illness, the prominence of depression has been noted, leading some early researchers to conclude that emotions were instrumental in causing the disease. In the literature over the past thirty years the argument has been raging: Is CFIDS an organic illness or a form of mental illness? Is depression the cause of CFIDS or a result of it?

Soon after the Lake Tahoe outbreak in 1985, the debate on the role of depression as the cause of CFIDS began in the United States, the same debate that had been raging in the thirty-five years since the Royal Free outbreak in London. Some physicians maintained that no illness was present at all, some that the symptoms were due to emotional disturbance, and some that an organic disease was causing emotional symptoms. When the name "yuppie flu" appeared, practicing physicians dismissed CFIDS, assuming it was either a hoax, mass hysteria, or simple depression. This dismissal of CFIDS as an unimportant or trivial illness developed further when the Epstein-Barr virus, which was once considered a hot lead, did not prove to be the causal agent. It is a tribute to the researchers studying patients in Incline Village that they persisted despite the medical pressure and censure they faced.

The argument has been bitter because of the conviction and insistence of patients that although emotional symptoms are present in the illness, a primary emotional disturbance is not its cause. Patients, patient support groups, and some researchers have pointed out the many factors that argue against mental illness. Patients are angry and frustrated, interpreting the debate over emotions as trivialization of their illness and as the explanation for why so little has been done to help them.

Patients who suggested to their physicians that CFIDS might be causing their symptoms were all too often greeted with a shrug of the shoulders, and "Oh, the yuppie business." And the diagnosis of depression may have been a convenient way of getting rid of these troublesome patients who complained all the time but had normal blood tests. By making the diagnosis of depression and referring a patient for psychiatric care, the primary care physician could write a diagnosis into the chart, one that theoretically answered the questions and relieved the doctor from further responsibilities.

But like so many aspects of medicine, the issues are not that simple. Within this diagnosis of depression there are numerous related disorders, ranging from an organic brain syndrome, clearly caused by organic factors, to malingering, commonly known as "faking it." The anger of so many patients has been at least partially due to their perception that physicians believe they are making up the symptoms.

The debate has raged among CFIDS researchers as well. Studies have documented the presence of depression, anxiety, and panic attacks in patients. Some researchers conclude from these studies that depression is the cause of CFIDS, while others state that the presence of emotional symptoms does not prove a psychiatric cause. I freely admit to my bias in this argument: I am among those who do not believe that depression or mental illness is the cause of CFIDS. Many patients with cancer are depressed, yet depression is not the cause of cancer. In medicine we refer to the role played by depression as being either primary or secondary.

Primary and Secondary Depression

Primary depression is a psychiatric illness that has been studied extensively for many years. Its hallmark and main symptoms are feelings of loss, despair, despondency, apathy, and sadness. Associated symptoms include fatigue, change in appetite, sleep disturbance, and sometimes agitation. Other symptoms sometimes seen include headaches and functional bowel problems. However, in primary depression the most dominant symptom is despair and hopelessness, and all other symptoms are relatively minor. Psychiatric evaluations may determine the cause or causes of these feelings, and with counseling and / or medication the symptoms improve.

The symptoms of primary depression are quite dissimilar to the symptoms of CFIDS patients. While up to 60 percent of patients are depressed, 40 percent are not, or have only minimal depression expected from the life disruption they experience. Emotionally healthy children develop CFIDS and have less depression than adults in this first few years of the illness. And perhaps the most impressive evidence is offered in the numerous reported outbreaks. If CFIDS is mental illness, why does it occur in epidemics? Mass hysteria is an inadequate answer because the symptoms of mass hysteria are random, whereas the pattern of symptoms in CFIDS is remarkably consistent. There is no explanation for the observed epidemiology if CFIDS is due to the minor stresses and strains of daily life.

Furthermore, numerous prominent symptoms of CFIDS are not associated with depression. Up to 75 percent of adult patients begin their illness with an acute illness similar to influenza or mononucleosis. No such association is common in primary depression. The symptoms of CFIDS include joint pain, visual disturbances, muscle pain, sore throat, lymphatic pain, fever, chills, night sweats, urinary frequency, paresthesias (numbness and tingling), and skin rash, none of which are traditionally felt to be symptoms of primary depression. Despair, hopelessness, and apathy are prominent in primary depression, but patients with CFIDS do not lack the desire to be active. Rather, they are depressed because they are physically unable to carry out normal activities.

Even the shared symptom of fatigue is different in the two illnesses. In primary depression, fatigue is secondary to inertia and lack of motivation. A patient with depression who does exercise usually feels refreshed, at least for a while. If a patient with CFIDS pushes himself or herself to exercise, the fatigue becomes worse, characterized by malaise, a sick, exhausted, and flulike feeling.

When CFIDS patients describe the depression they feel, they state that they had no emotional symptoms until some time after the appearance of exhaustion, muscle aches and other symptoms. They describe the depression as a result of their inability to carry on with normal activities, and of the disruption and pain caused by the many symptoms, a classic description of secondary depression. Added to this is the frustration of being unable to find an explanation for the symptoms they experience. The inability to establish a diagnosis merely increases the severity of the secondary depression.

Numerous illnesses are associated with secondary depression. For example, patients with malignancies are depressed for the obvious reason that their life is in danger. Secondary depression in patients with serious malignancies is so reasonable and expected that a patient without it would have his or her sanity questioned. Secondary depression is seen in multiple sclerosis, lupus, and virtually all other chronic illnesses.

Dysthymic disorder, sometimes called depressive neurosis, is a milder and more vague disturbance than major depression, and physicians may actually be referring to this condition when they state that CFIDS is emotional in origin. However, in dysthymia the diagnosis again revolves around feelings of hopelessness, poor self-esteem, and abnormal social situations. Organic symptoms such as sore throat and lymph node pain are not felt to be a part of this syndrome.

Primary depression is a common disorder, and it is quite likely that CFIDS patients have primary depression at least as often as the general public. It is also possible that depression causes minimal immunologic abnormalities and, like allergies, may be a risk factor for the development of CFIDS. If depression is found to be a risk factor for CFIDS, this does not mean that it is a cause of the illness.

*S*omatization and Malingering

Somatization disorder, also called Briquet's syndrome, is characterized by symptoms that suggest organ damage when in fact the symptoms are psychological (soma = body). The symptoms may be an exaggeration of a minor injury, or a set of vague, diffuse complaints that have no organic basis. The key to the diagnosis is that there is something the patient hopes to gain by being sick, such as attention, pity, or avoidance of responsibility. In somatization disorder, there is frequently a history of markedly abnormal personal relationships, often with physical violence, a history of neglect or abuse as a child, and substance abuse. It is not an easy diagnosis to make. In one series of patients diagnosed with somatization disorder, almost half were later found to have an organic disorder that could explain the symptoms. So much for the diagnostic accuracy of modern psychiatry.

Somatization is not under voluntary control, but malingering is. Simply put, malingering is making up symptoms in order to obtain something. For example, to make a million dollars in a lawsuit, a person claims to be unable to walk after an accident. Such people state that they are confined to a wheelchair, but when they are in their own house, they walk without difficulty. In this example there is no unconscious motive or desire to be sick; it is simply a matter of fraud and is consciously undertaken by the person pretending to be sick. It is a reason that private detectives are hired.

Patients with CFIDS are frequently devastated when their physician suggests a referral to a psychiatrist. The referral may be a genuine attempt to examine the complex symptoms or to evaluate whether counseling would help the patient in coping with the illness. However, often the patient hears the physician saying that the symptoms are not really there. This perceived accusation of fraud, as well as the reluctance of physicians to recognize that the pattern of symptoms exists, is why many patients have become so angry.

There is a simple way to prove that CFIDS is not somatization or malingering. With these two latter conditions there may be numerous variable symptoms, but they are random. In CFIDS the symptoms are not random—they form a specific pattern. The statistical odds of any two patients describing these numerous symptoms in an identical way are astronomical. Yet patient after patient describes the same symptom complex in CFIDS. The symptoms may appear random to physicians if they have not heard them before. Therefore, physicians must take the time to listen to the entire history. I have no doubt that any physician who does listen carefully will be convinced of the specificity of the symptoms of this syndrome very quickly. But a physician who spends only five minutes per visit will not perceive this pattern of symptoms, even after examining a hundred patients with CFIDS.

*B*iologic Depression

The separation of illnesses into either organic or psychiatric classifications has always been difficult for practicing physicians. In CFIDS, this task has been even more difficult because of the nature of the symptoms, the physical findings, and the normal routine laboratory results. However, five clues serve to indicate an organic rather than a psychiatric cause (Cecil *Textbook of Medicine*).

1. The signs and symptoms do not fit an established psychiatric diagnostic category.

2. The patient had no prior psychiatric history or symptoms.

3. The patient demonstrates an abrupt change in behavior or personality.

4. The signs and symptoms fluctuate rapidly.

5. The condition does not respond to psychiatric treatment.

According to these criteria, CFIDS is an organic and not a psychiatric disorder.

Many diseases of the brain are likely to have depression as a prominent symptom. In fact, there are organic causes of a whole range of emotional states, including anxiety, delirium, and even psychosis. Emotions are mediated by neurotransmitters (chemicals in the brain that transmit signals within and between neurons), and several areas of the brain are known to be particularly important in the regulation of emotions. At present we consider a disease with emotional symptoms to be organic if we know the medical or biologic cause, calling it an organic brain syndrome. There is a long list of disease states that have prominent organic depression, including vitamin B12 deficiency, hypothyroidism, brain tumors, and AIDS.

Drugs, medications, toxic exposures, and poisoning cause depression probably by altering the pattern or amounts of neurotransmitters. The list of drugs able to cause depression is extensive. Drugs and other chemicals are considered exogenous factors—they come from outside the body. That normal body chemicals, which may be increased in CFIDS, also cause depression is now of great interest to researchers.

As will be discussed in a later chapter, chemicals known as cytokines, made by the healthy immune system, can cause depression. Two of the best-studied cytokines are alpha interferon and interleukin-2. Hints are now being found that these cytokines may be involved in generating the symptoms of CFIDS. This represents a possible breakthrough in the understanding not only of CFIDS but of mental illness as well.

*A*nxiety Disorders

Like depression, anxiety disorders are common and may have symptoms that mimic medical illnesses. Prominent symptoms include feelings of panic, anxiety, flushing, shortness of breath, chest pains, palpitations, headache, and gastrointestinal disturbances. All of these symptoms are prominent in CFIDS and, as in depression, give rise to the question: Is CFIDS merely a manifestation of an anxiety state, or is an anxiety state one of the symptoms of CFIDS?

Much of the previous discussion on depression can be applied to anxiety states. There are numerous medical causes for anxiety, including heart disease, asthma, and hyperthyroidism. Like depression, anxiety states are mediated by the body's biochemistry and neurotransmitters. For the same reasons as discussed in the preceding paragraphs, anxiety states are probably a symptom of CFIDS, and not the cause.

CFIDS patients often state that relapses (worsening of symptoms) occur with periods of stress. Some patients have even related the acute onset of the illness to an episode of severe stress. Avoidance of stress is a standard part of treatment, but even when patients quit their jobs in an attempt to avoid stress, the symptoms do not go away. Stress aggravates symptoms but does not cause them, a condition no different in CFIDS from that in other illnesses. Walking on a twisted ankle may aggravate the pain but did not cause the twisted ankle originally.

It is obvious that anxiety and depression are intertwined with chronic fatigue / immune dysfunction syndrome. That inappropriate diagnoses of primary emotional disorder have caused so much pain for those with CFIDS, contributing to the mistrust and anger of patients, is unfortunate. It has become such a sensitive subject that patients may grow angry when researchers even attempt to explore this link, a link that nearly all agree exists. CFIDS is an illness that affects the brain and the immune system. It causes depression, anxiety, and panic attacks in addition to its many physical symptoms.

In the early days of AIDS, emotions were blamed for causing the illness. Yet a cause was eventually found that explained the entire range of findings, including the emotional symptoms. Once the practicing physician becomes familiar with the symptom pattern of CFIDS, the emotional symptoms need no longer be seen as a simple explanation of the illness. The emotional symptoms will become a part of this larger pattern and ultimately contribute to understanding the cause.

*A*llergies

One of the first associations made with CFIDS was the presence of multiple allergies and chemical sensitivities. This association has been important for several reasons. Originally it became one of the arguments that CFIDS could not be hypochondriasis because a statistical association would not be possible in a random fabrication of symptoms. It also initiated hypotheses concerning a shared mechanism within the immune system. The association with allergies also serves to imply a genetic predisposition for the illness, and this can help to predict who may be at risk for developing CFIDS.

Allergy plays a role in CFIDS in two ways: people who develop this illness are likely to have a history of allergies prior to becoming ill, and allergies may develop for the first time with the onset of CFIDS. Numerous scientific papers have noted the association between CFIDS and allergies, although studies on the mechanisms are more rare.

Simply stated, allergies are an immunological response to a substance or substances that would normally cause the body no harm. Hay fever is an example of a typical allergy. In this condition, pollen is inhaled and settles on the lining of the airways. In a person without allergies, this event goes unnoticed except for the cells that clear away debris. However, in the allergic person, the event is met with an immune response (up-regulation) that resembles an attempt to fight an infection. The body misinterprets the pollen and treats the allergen as if it were an invading bacteria or virus. Antibodies are manufactured and cellular chemicals are released, causing runny nose, sneezing, and sometimes wheezing.

The tendency of some people to develop allergies has a genetic basis, and thus allergies may serve as a genetic marker. If both parents have allergies, a child has nearly a 75 percent chance of developing allergies during his or her lifetime. If neither parent has allergies, the risk is much lower, slightly more than 10 percent. Specific allergies are not inherited, but the tendency toward allergies is. This is known as genetic predisposition.

It is possible that because of a genetic predisposition to allergy, some people are more likely to develop CFIDS than others, even if both are exposed to the same underlying cause of CFIDS. While not proving that CFIDS is a form of allergy, it would account for studies showing a prior history of allergy. CFIDS also has a high incidence in certain families, again implying a genetic predisposition.

Many patients who had childhood allergies and were free of them for many years develop allergies again when they become ill with CFIDS. And some patients who have never had allergies at all will develop them after becoming ill. Of course, some patients with CFIDS have no allergic symptoms; therefore, the presence of allergies is not required to make the diagnosis of CFIDS. CFIDS is not exclusively an allergic disease, and the increased incidence merely reflects an association.

Allergies can be thought of as an up-regulated immune response—a gun with a hair trigger. Minor, nonthreatening events can initiate the allergic reaction, and this reaction is inappropriate. As will be discussed in a later section on immunology, CFIDS may also be an up-regulated immune response. With allergies we are usually able to detect the culprit; skin tests may show an exaggerated response to pollen, for example. But with CFIDS we do not know why the immune system seems to be working overtime. This shared mechanism probably accounts for the similarities between the two illnesses.

Unfortunately, standard allergy treatments are of little help in CFIDS. Many people have had an extensive series of desensitization shots—allergy shots—with little benefit. This poor result is because we are probably not addressing the specific cause of the immune activation in CFIDS. One interesting hypothesis is that rather than a benign substance such as pollen, the offending agent in CFIDS is an infectious agent, such as a virus. This would explain both the outbreaks of CFIDS and the immune system activation.

Although numerous infectious agents have been examined, none has been found to explain this association. An infectious cause of allergy has been questioned for years, and we know that some virus infections are associated with hives, also considered to be an allergic phenomenon. Yet the culprit responsible for CFIDS remains elusive. If an infectious agent is responsible for the association between CFIDS and allergy, it is likely to be a previously unknown agent.

Chemical Sensitivities

Sensitivities to chemicals and odors are considered to be in a separate class from true allergies because they are not mediated by the same immunologic mechanisms. There is considerable discussion as to what actually causes chemical sensitivities, but most researchers agree that they also involve immune system activation. Patients with chemical sensitivities as their most debilitating symptoms are said to have environmental allergy or chemical sensitivity syndrome. However, these symptoms are frequently seen in CFIDS, usually in a mild form, and the symptoms are elicited only by direct questioning. It is my feeling that in patients with severe chemical sensitivities who also have the symptoms of exhaustion, joint and muscle pain, headache, sore throat, and abdominal discomfort, CFIDS probably is the cause of the chemical sensitivities.

CFIDS patients with chemical sensitivities have an added burden because of the limitations these symptoms place on them. If the level of exhaustion and other symptoms is relatively minor, the sensitivities may be the reason they are unable to function at their job. These sensitivities can be completely disabling, since the range of odors and sensitizing agents is enormous. A new rug, cologne, perfume on a friend, gasoline odors in a car, dust or odors in a factory—all can cause exacerbation of the symptoms of CFIDS.

Unlike multiple allergies, of which most patients have preexisting symptoms, patients with chemical sensitivities usually develop them months to years after first experiencing CFIDS. The existence of severe chemical sensitivities appears to be greatest in those who have had CFIDS for more than five to ten years, and it is relatively rare to see it in the first year of the illness.

Ultimately, the treatment for allergic symptoms in CFIDS will revolve around either the elimination of the underlying cause of the illness or a safe way of dampening the overactive immune response. Unfortunately, neither of these approaches is successful at the present time.

*F*ibromyalgia

Fibromyalgia is a condition characterized by painful aching of the muscles. The illness is associated with numerous other symptoms, including fatigue, cognitive difficulties, sleep disturbance, joint pain, headache, and abdominal pain. It may occur secondarily to several disease states, such as rheumatoid arthritis or lupus erythematosis, or it may be isolated, in which case it is called primary fibromyalgia.

One current controversy among researchers is whether primary fibromyalgia is the same illness as CFIDS. Although nearly all CFIDS patients have muscle pain, many do not have enough muscle pain to elicit the tender points on examination, the basis of the fibromyalgia diagnosis. However, the overall pattern of symptoms is strikingly similar. The discussion has not yet been resolved, but I think it is likely that CFIDS and primary fibromyalgia are the same illness.

One caution for patients with chronic fatigue: it is a mistake to assume that all fatigue is due to CFIDS. People with chronic fatigue need a complete and careful medical evaluation. For those who have CFIDS, the diagnosis should be reviewed on a regular basis. I urge CFIDS patients to have a complete physical examination at least once yearly, including complete cancer screening as recommended by the American Cancer Society. Patients with CFIDS may develop other illnesses, and careful medical reevaluation with this in mind is appropriate.

*C*onclusion

Understanding the relationship of CFIDS to other diseases will be a long and difficult task. At present, we must rely on symptoms, and symptoms may be shared by different illnesses. It is likely that this task will not be accomplished until the cause of CFIDS is known. Until then, we are forced to rely on whatever hints are available to us.

CHAPTER 4

CFIDS and Children

Chronic fatigue / immune dysfunction syndrome has received most attention in the description of its devastating effects on previously healthy and productive adults. But the disorder also affects children, and the consequences may be equally devastating. What follows is a fictionalized account of the havoc CFIDS can wreak on children.

Kevin Jennings—A Case History

November 4 had been an unbelievable day, one in a million. Sixteen-year-old Kevin Jennings, in his junior year of high school, had been elected co-captain of next year's soccer team and named to the all-state squad, both on the same day. An honor roll student, he was beginning to think of applying to colleges known for their soccer teams. And with his grades, he might even get a scholarship.

It was Tuesday afternoon—he had been looking forward to celebrating that afternoon at the team practice, but his mother had scheduled an appointment for him with Dr. Ashford, their pediatrician. Kevin had been having dizzy spells and headaches—a minor annoyance, but there was no way he could get out of the appointment.

Kevin was bored waiting in the doctor's office. There were many things he would rather be doing. He had been having headaches almost daily for weeks, but they were mild and did not interfere with his activities. Usually he would take two aspirin and the headache would disappear. The dizzy spells were more annoying, but they were not severe, and he wished he had not even mentioned them to his mother. He sat through the examination patiently while Dr. Ashford peered into his eyes and ears with a bright light. The light hurt his eyes. Other than a blister in his mouth, which didn't bother him, the examination was normal.

Believing that Kevin's symptoms were due to labyrinthitis, a viral infection of the inner ear and balance center, Dr. Ashford prescribed an antihistamine. Kevin wanted to rejoin the team practice, but by the time his appointment was over it was too late. The team had made the sectional playoffs, and the first game would be this coming Saturday.

Two days later Kevin became ill. He had a severe sore throat, painful swollen glands in his neck, and a fever of 103°. He was exhausted and was unable to eat because of nausea. He spent the day in bed, hoping that he would be better by Saturday.

But by Saturday he was no better, and although he dressed for the game, he was unable to play. Kevin did not object to sitting on the bench, for he was so exhausted that he could barely walk. The team they were playing was the best in the state, and Kevin's team lost by three goals. The season was over. There was always next year.

Kevin stayed home from school on Monday and slept the entire day. He had developed pain in his stomach in both right and left sides under his ribs. He still had a sore throat and ached all over. His joints, especially his knees and wrists, were sore. His mother made an appointment with Dr. Ashford for the next day.

Dr. Ashford felt that Kevin probably had strep throat and prescribed penicillin after taking a throat culture. He said that Kevin's spleen was a little enlarged, but Mrs. Jennings was relieved that it wasn't appendicitis. There was no obvious swelling in any of the joints. Kevin's dizzy spells and headaches were a little worse than before, but he forgot to mention this.

Three days later he returned to the physician's office because there had been no improvement. The strep test had been negative, and the penicillin had been of no value. On examination Dr. Ashford noticed that the lymph nodes in the armpit and groin were swollen and tender, just like the lymph nodes in the neck. Kevin's muscles ached, and his abdomen was still very tender in the liver and spleen area.

Dr. Ashford suspected that he had acute mononucleosis caused by the Epstein-Barr virus, and the pain in the liver area was most likely a hepatitis caused by mono. He ordered a complete blood count, a monospot to detect mononucleosis, and chemistries to detect hepatitis. The penicillin was stopped, and Kevin would have to stay in bed for the next two weeks because mono frequently goes on that long. The doctor would reexamine him in one week.

Kevin slept almost the entire week. There was no change in his symptoms, except that the fever was now lower than before. Another week passed. And another. Kevin had been out of school for a month, and he showed no signs of getting better, although the mono test had come back negative.

Exhaustion was the only symptom that never varied from day to day. It seemed that every day a different symptom was making him feel sick. One day the headaches were severe, with lymph pain and stomach ache less prominent. The next day it was the sore throat and muscle aching that was most severe. The next day, dizzy spells and racing heartbeat. The next day, joint pain.

Dr. Ashford, completely bewildered, was becoming frustrated. He ordered more tests on every visit until Kevin thought he would run out of blood. All the routine counts and chemistries were normal, as were X rays, liver function, and thyroid tests. Epstein-Barr virus antibodies, more sensitive than the monospot, were done and showed that Kevin had never had the virus. There was no chance that this illness had anything to do with the virus that usually causes mono. Antibodies for Lyme disease, toxoplasmosis, cytomegalovirus, parasites, rickettsia, and other mysterious infections were negative.

Dr. Ashford decided to approach the problem system by system. For the abdominal pain, an upper and lower GI series and pancreatic sonogram were negative. For the headaches, a CT scan of his brain was negative. For the joint pain, rheumatoid arthritis and lupus tests were negative. And so on. Kevin thought it unlikely that there were any tests invented that had not been run. Then Dr. Ashford mentioned surgery.

One afternoon, when Kevin and his parents were in Dr. Ashford's office, the subject of cancer was brought up. Dr. Ashford began to talk about the possibility that Kevin's symptoms could be due to a malignancy. He worried about a lymphoma, or cancer of the lymph glands; he described how it was possible for this type of cancer to cause fevers and other symptoms, yet it could be hard to detect. They discussed and agreed on a lymph node biopsy. In a way, Mrs. Jennings was relieved, because she had begun to suspect something serious. Kevin agreed to the biopsy but seemed apathetic. When the results came back, they were negative once again.

Three months later Kevin was still sick. It was now April, and he had not been to school since November; no one had any idea of what was making him so ill. One of the many specialists Dr. Ashford had sent him to had suggested that Kevin was making up the symptoms, for they fit the pattern of no known disease and were too numerous.

But his symptoms hadn't changed much since the beginning. They were not as intense as before, but they were more constant, with less fluctuation. The fevers had gone, but not the night sweats. The sore throat, headache, lymph pain, stomach pain, and muscle and joint pain persisted. Kevin had dizzy spells, his heart would race, and he had occasional chest pain. And he had developed two new symptoms: A face rash appeared almost every day but was of minor significance. The other was more ominous—he could no longer think clearly or remember things.

About three months after first becoming ill it was obvious to Kevin that something was happening to his ability to think and reason. He had had difficulty earlier but attributed it to his tiredness and general feeling of malaise. One day when he was trying to say the word "truck," while talking to a friend, he could not say it, despite knowing what he wanted to say. Instead the word "tractor" came out. He turned it into a joke and ignored it, but after it began happening more often he knew he was losing his mind.

Attempts at home schooling and tutoring were unsuccessful. He felt poorly and slept much of the day, and he was unable to read or concentrate on his work. Several tutors came and went in frustration. One tutor said that Kevin was only pretending to be unable to read, and made a report to the school.

But for Kevin reading was just impossible. He would sit there, and his eyes ached as he tried to focus on the page. Lights hurt his eyes, which felt dry and scratchy. He had seen an eye specialist, but there was no explanation for his blurry vision. He struggled to follow the words across the page, but they made little sense. He would become lost in the middle of paragraphs, and at the end of a paragraph he had no idea of what he had read.

He had seen the school psychologist on several occasions and the school physician once. They had letters from Dr. Ashford saying that Kevin's absence was due to an undiagnosed medical illness, but they also had reports from other specialists who maintained that there was nothing medically wrong and that perhaps some psychological factors might be responsible. The tutor's report suggested that Kevin's problems were entirely psychological. The school psychologist had no doubt that the whole illness had been nonsense. He made a report to the superintendent of schools that Kevin should be made to attend school: his problem was school phobia, and the treatment was to attend school no matter how much he didn't want to.

Kevin's parents did not believe that he could have developed a psychological problem so suddenly, especially school phobia, since he was doing so well and had been so successful in school. But if he did not attend he would fail the year, and medical excuses would no longer be accepted. There was nothing Dr. Ashford could do.

Kevin's behavior had changed, however. Before last November he had been a relaxed and confident teenager. Now he seemed very anxious and was frequently having panic attacks for no apparent reason. At other times he would seem depressed and withdrawn. He discouraged his friends from coming to the house and visiting him. He sat in his room most of the day, doing little except watching television.

He was no longer seeing Dr. Ashford or any of the other physicians. His family was having severe financial problems because many of the medical bills were not covered by insurance. Some of the tests were not covered because the insurance company felt that there had been no medical reason to do them. All of the testing had been normal, even the lymph node biopsy, yet Dr. Ashford did not believe that Kevin's illness was psychological.

For two days Kevin went to school. He tried to act as if nothing was wrong and sat through classes that meant nothing to him. He had obviously fallen way behind, but in addition it was as if the classes were being taught in a foreign language. Between classes he walked slowly in the hallways, his head spinning, feeling off balance and totally exhausted. He saw the school psychologist, who thought that Kevin did not look very ill.

Kevin had noticed over the past three months that when he tried to exert himself he would get much worse. After spending three days lying in bed he would improve to the point where he could get up and walk around the house. And almost invariably he would do something strenuous, like going out to the backyard and throwing the basketball through the hoop. Then the symptoms would become worse.

His two days in school were a disaster, and, as he had feared, he had a major relapse. He began running a fever, and his joints, which had recently been fairly quiet, began hurting. He developed a severe sore throat, and increased pain in the lymph nodes and abdomen, and was so exhausted that he was unable to get out of bed even for meals. It seemed clear that he would have to fail the year at school.

Early the next week a social worker from the county child protective services came to the door. Kevin was truant from school without a medical reason, and the school physician had reported Kevin's family for child abuse. The charge was neglect for not requiring him to attend school. Kevin lay in bed while his parents fought with the social worker. A lawyer was hired and more physicians were consulted. Months passed, and eventually the judge dropped the charges of child abuse against Kevin's family because Dr. Ashford had written a letter stating that while the exact cause of Kevin's illness was unknown, he did not have school phobia or emotional problems. Kevin's parents had begun reading everything they could find about medical research and unusual diseases.

Kevin had been ill for almost one year when the family heard of an immunologist doing research on chronic fatigue / immune dysfunction syndrome, or CFIDS. They visited the physician, and after taking a history and physical examination he ordered more blood tests, this time ones specific to the immune system. Skin tests showed decreased responses to common antigens, and the interleukin-2 receptor and alpha interferon levels were both elevated. Detailed studies of natural killer cells showed that both the concentration and the ability to react were abnormal. There was a depression of the number of T suppressor lymphocytes and a mild increase in B lymphocytes, something called polyclonal activation. The immunologist concluded that on the basis of a typical history, physical examination, and pattern of immune abnormalities, Kevin had CFIDS.

Neither Kevin nor his parents had a very good understanding of what these immunological tests meant. The immunologist explained that in CFIDS, the immune system appeared to be responding as if it were fighting a viral infection. The responses seen here were different from the responses seen in emotional illness. He wrote a letter to Dr. Ashford, the school, the school psychologist, and other referring physicians about Kevin's case. He tried a few medications that had immunoreactive properties, but they did little good.

But at least Kevin now had a diagnosis and he knew what was causing him to be ill. His symptoms, prolonged course, and immunological profile were due to CFIDS. No one at the school really believed him, certainly not the school psychologist, who fumed that Kevin had been able to "pull it off" by finding some quack physician who had told him what he wanted to hear. Dr. Ashford had not heard of this disease before and did not know how to interpret the immunological tests. But he had known all along that something was medically wrong with Kevin. And it was his support that Kevin appreciated as much as the immunologist's research on CFIDS.

A Child's Symptoms

As can be seen by Kevin's case, CFIDS does not limit itself to
adults. Although some children have atypical presentations, the
discussion here will focus on children who have a typical clinical
presentation. Because of special problems involving child development, the diagnosis of CFIDS in children may be difficult or impossible to make using the definition offered by the Centers for
Disease Control (Holmes 88). I prefer to make the diagnosis using
a modification of these criteria based on the presence of chronic
fatigue and a characteristic pattern of symptoms:

1. Chronic fatigue
    At least 50% reduction in overall activity for six months

2. Symptom pattern
    At least 8 of the 12 following symptoms:
        Malaise
        Sleep disorder
        Headache
        Recurrent sore throat
        Lymph node pain
        Muscle pain
        Joint pain
        Abdominal pain
        Eye pain / light sensitivity
        Neurocognitive (attention / short-term memory)
        Balance disturbance / paresthesias / dizziness /
            light-headedness
        Temperature regulatory symptoms (fever / chills / night
            sweats)

3. Absence of other disease process to explain symptom complex

In general, the symptom pattern in children is similar to that
in adults, but there are a few exceptions. One striking difference
is that in children the numerous symptoms appear to be almost
equally severe. In adults it is common to hear that certain symptoms are always the most severe, but children may state that sore

throat and headaches are the worst symptom one day, followed the next day by lymphatic and abdominal pain. This rotation of symptoms is frustrating, for just when the pediatrician is about to begin an evaluation of the headaches, they may improve, replaced by joint pains as the most severe symptom.

The variation in symptoms and their intensity is the primary reason for the frequent misdiagnosis of emotional disorder, particularly school phobia. However, these diagnoses require the presence of a secondary gain for the diagnosis to be acceptable. That is, children who invent somatic symptoms do so because there is something they wish to gain, and which they can achieve by being "sick." Sometimes the only way a child can achieve the attention of the parents is by being sick; illness allows him or her to gain love, sympathy, and attention.

In school phobia, children do not want to go to school, usually because of fear of separation from the parents, and they will invent ways to avoid it. Therefore, because of the anxiety about going to school, a child might have a stomachache and not "feel well" at 7:30 on a school-day morning. But these complaints are never expressed in the afternoon, when school is over, or on Saturday morning.

The evaluation of behavior disorders in children is directed toward looking for these secondary gains, and they are usually easy to find. But in CFIDS, there are no significant secondary gains; the symptoms are equally present on nonschool days, and play activity is impaired. If an important secondary gain is present on family interview, the diagnosis of CFIDS in children should not be made unless the symptoms persist after the secondary gain is removed.

Another difference between adults and children exists in the neurologic symptoms. Adults have a clear perception of their abilities, so that memory loss and inability to concentrate are easily recognized. Children are less sure of their abilities, and these symptoms manifest as progressive school difficulties. Dizziness and light-headedness are common symptoms in children. Seizure disorders, particularly atypical petit mal seizures, are more common than in adults. Overall, the neurologic symptoms in children are less debilitating than in adults, but because they occur during a period of rapid learning and intellectual development, the long-term problems generated by these symptoms may be greater.

There appear to be two general patterns of CFIDS in children, those with a gradual or insidious onset of symptoms, usually occurring in children five to twelve years of age, and those with an acute onset of symptoms, usually during adolescence. For the purpose of simplicity, I define acute onset as a sudden appearance of symptoms within a few days to weeks, usually a flulike illness in a child who had previously been entirely well. The gradual appearance of symptoms over several months or longer, or the presence of mild symptoms suggestive of CFIDS prior to an acute episode, would be defined as an insidious onset. These two types of presentation will be treated separately because they present separate diagnostic and management problems. Although we will be linking acute onset with older children and insidious onset with younger children, there is considerable crossover.

Acute Onset During Adolescence

The majority, perhaps 75 percent, of children that can be diagnosed with CFIDS fall into this category. Because of special difficulties in making the diagnosis in younger children, however, this percentage could be inaccurate. At the present stage of research, it is probably wise to restrict definition of CFIDS to those in whom the diagnosis is indisputable, and as our knowledge increases, more precise diagnosis of atypical presentations will become possible.

The diagnosis of CFIDS in the adolescent is very similar to that in the adult. The majority seem to be healthy growing children who have a flulike or mononucleosis-like illness and then persist with symptoms for months or years. The most prominent symptoms are fatigue, headache, abdominal pain, joint and muscle pain, eye pain, dizziness, and lymphatic pain.

The diagnosis of CFIDS in children with acute onset is the same as for the adult. These children are articulate and can clearly state their symptoms, such as degree of fatigue, cognitive difficulties, and degree of activity impairment. Their school problems can be traced to the onset of the illness, because they have already established learning patterns. Social and behavioral problems may be compared to their preillness state.

These children may accumulate a bewildering array of diagnoses, but there is less diagnostic confusion than with children with insidious onset. Other diagnoses that may be confused with CFIDS include childhood migraine syndrome, Crohn's disease, atypical epilepsy, school phobia, attention deficit disorder, ankylosing spondylitis, rheumatoid arthritis, chronic rheumatic fever, functional abdominal pain, food allergy syndrome, and numerous others.

Insidious Onset in the Younger Child

I have rarely seen a sudden acute onset of CFIDS in a child younger than ten years old. Children from five to ten have a gradual onset of symptoms, with periods when certain symptoms become more prominent. It may be that a child presents after a flulike illness with symptoms suggestive of CFIDS, but questioning often reveals that the child has had frequent sore throats, headaches, or joint pains, and has been relatively inactive, sleeping more than other children of the same age. None of these children would be diagnosed as having CFIDS by the Centers for Disease Control diagnostic criteria because they lack a new onset of fatigue. Because the onset of fatigue may be impossible to date, this criterion cannot be fulfilled. Children with a gradual onset of symptoms are often not able to articulate the precise degree of fatigue, nor are they able to describe cognitive difficulties because they may not have experienced a time period without them.

Do these children really have CFIDS? This is a difficult question to answer, mainly because the degree of severity of their symptoms appears less than the acute onset adolescent. Young children who grow up with symptoms of CFIDS have become accustomed to the symptoms and are able to function well despite persistent and sometimes severe discomfort.

Our office research staff examined the symptomatology of twenty children between the ages of five and twelve who had a gradual onset of their symptoms, and compared them to the symptoms of the same number of adolescents with acute onset of CFIDS roughly one year after onset. With the exception of the degree of disability, there was no way to tell the difference between these two groups. The incidence of fatigue, headache, joint pain, muscle pain, sore throat, eye pain, and other symptoms was identical. However, children with acute onset during adolescence were clearly more ill in the first six months after the onset of their illness. The difference in degree of severity became less prominent as months passed.

Children with early insidious onset frequently do not perceive themselves as being ill, most likely because they have been growing up with the symptoms. Children with acute onset perceived themselves as ill and had missed more days of school. It was difficult to decide by objective criteria which group was more ill. When laboratory parameters become more firmly established, it will be interesting to compare these groups.

*S*chool Disorders

Children with CFIDS have problems in several developmental areas, frequently causing school failure. In a series of thirty-two children diagnosed with CFIDS (Bell 89), all but one child had worsening of school performance, with 70 percent having their average grade level fall by two grades or more. Of these children, 66 percent described their problems as "severe," 3 percent as "moderate," and 25 percent as "mild"; only 6 percent described no school problems. Of the twenty-one children with severe school problems, twelve missed more than six months of school, eight missed between three and six months of school, and only one missed less than three months.

Numerous factors are involved in the difficulties faced by the school-age child with CFIDS, including severity of the illness, time lost from school, the degree of cognitive problems (ability to think clearly), the flexibility of the educational program, family functioning, and the child's ability to cope. Perhaps the most important factor in school difficulty is the severity of CFIDS. Although no one knows the entire spectrum of illness in the school-age child, it appears that the range is between almost normal activity and no obvious cognitive difficulties to children who are bedridden with severe cognitive impairment. All grades of disability exist, and the degree of impairment usually fluctuates with time.

The two major patterns of CFIDS in children are reflected in the pattern of school problems. For children with acute onset the difficulties are similar to those with any acute illness in the first few months. A previously well and healthy child has the acute onset of CFIDS, and time is lost from school because of illness and diagnostic measures. After the medical issues have been clarified, a period of adjustment occurs when many children begin to resume their school work, hopefully with appropriate changes in academic schedule or even home tutoring. The subsequent course is similar to other prolonged illnesses.

The gradual onset is more difficult to assess. The symptoms of CFIDS appear at an early age in an insidious manner, with no episodes of acute illness. After fruitless visits to physicians, no diagnosis or explanation of the symptoms is offered, leaving the family and school with the incorrect impression that no organic illness exists. Occasionally, a diagnosis of learning disability, behavior disorder, or school phobia is made. With these children less time is lost from school because the fatigue is not as severe, but the child is not functioning at full capacity while attending school.

For both onset patterns the cognitive symptoms include loss of ability to concentrate, difficulties in short-term memory and word-finding ability, and difficulties in visual/spatial perception. The most common is the inability to maintain attention. This is reflected in difficulties with reading or reading comprehension. Children, like adults, state that they become lost while in the middle of a paragraph or during an explanation. The degree of this loss of concentration seems to parallel the degree of fatigue and may be a general phenomenon rather than a specific cognitive defect. These problems in children with gradual or insidious onset are more likely to go unrecognized, because these children can be considered complainers and are not perceived as being sick. There appears to be considerable variation in the degree of cognitive difficulties, although specific studies to look at this area have not been done. While some bright students may spontaneously develop "tricks" to help them get around certain cognitive difficulties, it goes without saying that after a child develops CFIDS, he or she must work harder to maintain the same grades.

Emotional Disorders

The family struggling with CFIDS must function well. There needs to be good communication between parent and child, appropriate behavior control, and above all, trust. The parents must be able to accurately assess the degree of impairment caused by illness and when secondary behavior problems occur. This is difficult in any chronic childhood illness, but especially so in CFIDS. Just as a child with juvenile rheumatoid arthritis may begin to manipulate the family, behavior problems in a child with CFIDS occur and must be approached in a consistent and firm manner. Counseling with an expert in child behavior may be of value in separating the various factors.

In the study of thirty-two children previously cited, an attempt was made to assess the degree of family and emotional difficulty. Only four study subjects or their parents (12.5 percent) felt that family relationships and functioning were unaffected by the symptoms. Of the remaining twenty-eight children, "mild" problems were described in twenty (62.5 percent), "moderate" in seven (21.9 percent), and "severe" in one (3.1 percent). The most common problems described related to poor communication, stresses revolving around school absences, and inability to participate in family activities. One difficulty frequently stated as contributing to family disturbance was the frustration generated by the inability to define a cause for the symptoms.

Only four of these thirty-two children (12.5 percent) described no social problems on questioning. "Mild" problems were described in thirteen (40.6 percent), "moderate" in six (18.8 percent), and "severe" in twelve (37.5 percent). The more severe social and interactive difficulties were present in boys unable to participate in sports at the same level as they had prior to becoming ill.

The greatest concern about children who develop CFIDS at an early age is the possibility of an increased chance that symptoms will persist indefinitely. Numerous adults with a longstanding history of CFIDS date the onset of their symptoms to childhood, and it may be less common for acute onset adults to have persistence of symptoms. Studies examining this suspicion have not been done.

In later chapters we will discuss the possibility that the symptoms of CFIDS are due to an abnormal immune response. Because of differences in the immune response of adults and children, it is possible that the flexibility of the child's immune response permits less severity of symptoms while at the same time increasing the likelihood of persistence of symptoms. If this proves correct, then children with CFIDS are at far greater risk for long-term emotional and physical disability than adults.

Conclusion

There are probably few illnesses in which the need for an accurate diagnosis is more important than in CFIDS. Although diagnosis may not prevent medical complications, and may not always offer relief of symptoms, it is essential for healthy emotional development and long-range educational planning. The reason is simple: the symptoms of CFIDS are frequently perceived by medical and school personnel as school phobia, emotional disorder, lack of motivation, laziness, or lack of effort on the part of the child. Failure to establish the diagnosis, and lack of cooperation between professionals, may lead to inaccurate impressions of malingering on the part of the child, with subsequent isolation, insecurity, sense of failure, family stress, and even legal action against the family by school authorities. Prevention of these difficulties can be achieved with accurate diagnosis.

PART 3

The Tests

CHAPTER 5

Laboratory Evaluation in CFIDS

As we have seen, a large part of the tragedy of CFIDS is the difficulty in diagnosis. Sufferers often find themselves pulled into what seems to be an endless array of tests, each one coming back negative, until many would feel relief if something, anything, came back positive. The purpose of this section is to explain the need for all these tests, as well as to serve as a guide through the often bewildering maze of the medical world that CFIDS patients become all too intimately acquainted with.

The laboratory evaluation in CFIDS has been an exceedingly difficult topic for several reasons. Physicians have been confused because simple tests are not diagnostic, and have had difficulty deciding on the degree of exclusionary testing necessary. Moreover, they have been bewildered by the role of antibody testing for the Epstein-Barr virus. Worse yet, the tests that appear to be of greatest value in CFIDS—sophisticated and expensive tests of immunologic function—are not well understood by the majority of practicing physicians. Therefore, even when these tests are performed and the values are abnormal, they are greeted with a blank expression, as if to say, "Now, what does this mean?"

I think that the degree of a patient workup depends on two factors: the severity of CFIDS in an individual, and the economic resources and/or medical insurance coverage that the patient has. This latter factor is inexcusable in a civilized society, but it is a reality. The cost of a complete laboratory evaluation can be staggering. A patient without medical insurance, struggling to stay at work, and just able to make ends meet economically may be handed a laboratory bill of $7,000 for extensive blood tests and diagnostic procedures that add nothing to the clinical diagnosis. Yet from a legal standpoint, physicians are under great pressure to order numerous tests to explain the symptoms and to protect against what they perceive is the threat of future lawsuits.

A middle road is practical for most patients with CFIDS. If a patient has mild symptoms, an extensive workup is not necessary, and the appropriate laboratory evaluation should consist of excluding common illnesses that could cause fatigue. If a patient is severely ill, a more thorough evaluation is called for. A physician must exercise good common sense and clinical judgment in deciding on the most valuable and cost-effective tests to order.

There are several areas of laboratory evaluation possible for a patient with CFIDS: (a) exclusion of other illnesses that can produce fatigue and similar symptoms; (b) documentation of the process of viral reactivation and; (c) evaluation of the competence of the immune system. Documentation of the degree of disability, although not technically a laboratory test, will also be discussed at the end of this section.

It must be stressed that no single test or combination of tests is diagnostic for CFIDS. The diagnosis rests on a typical pattern of symptoms and exclusion of other causes of fatigue. Etiologic testing, looking for the cause of CFIDS, is not available at the time of this writing. The ultimate or perfect test would be one that measures the cause or causes of CFIDS, our Agent X, and this is not known. Such studies may be possible in the near future, and a simple diagnostic test may then solve the question of laboratory evaluation. Until this perfect test is found, we must be content with a more complex route.

The paragraphs that follow outline what I consider to be an appropriate basic laboratory evaluation for an individual with moderately severe CFIDS and offer a brief explanation of what these tests look for. This is a general discussion only, and patients with CFIDS or suggestive symptoms should consult their own physicians for opinions specific to their condition. Moreover, there may be as many approaches to the laboratory evaluation of CFIDS as there are physicians who study the illness. Even six months from now the evaluation may be quite different, but for the moment the following should be a useful synthesis for patients who may be overwhelmed with the barrage of medical terms they may never have heard before.

*E*xclusionary Tests

Laboratory tests in this category are performed to rule out other illnesses that can cause symptoms suggestive of CFIDS. Although I feel that the symptom pattern is specific for CFIDS, a thousand other illnesses may share some of this symptom pattern. It is obviously not necessary to test for all one thousand of these illnesses, but certain ones need to be considered and excluded. The tests I believe to be most useful and cost effective in accomplishing this task are listed below.

Complete Blood Count (CBC)

A complete blood count is a measure of the number of red blood cells and white blood cells and a differential count of what types of white blood cells are present. Probably every person who has seen a physician has had this standard test done. In CFIDS the complete blood count is usually normal and eliminates many illnesses, such as anemia. Occasionally, in patients with CFIDS, the while blood cell count is low, and this may imply the presence of a persistent viral infection. However, the count is not so low that patients are at risk for secondary infections.

The complete blood count may be strikingly abnormal in many illnesses with symptoms milder than CFIDS. Abscesses, blood disorders, certain malignancies, and other disorders may head to abnormal complete blood counts. But patients frequently are dismayed that despite feeling so poorly, their CBC is normal. The CBC is not an overall portrait of health.

Sedimentation Rate (Sed Rate)

This primitive test consists of letting a tube of blood sit on a counter for one hour and measuring the amount of separation between the blood cells and the fluid. It is like watching cream separate from milk, certainly not sophisticated, but useful nonetheless. Most serious illnesses have an elevated sed rate, and although it is not specific, physicians use it to separate disease states from normal. It has been said that if the sed rate is normal, nothing could be wrong with the patient. This has been one of the difficult hurdles that CFIDS patients face, for although they feel terrible, the sed rate is usually normal. I feel it is the single most useful test in diagnosis and management of CFIDS.

The normal range of sed rate is from 10 mm per hour to about 30 mm per hour. In CFIDS the sed rate is rarely elevated above 30 (Salit 85; Buchwald 87) and in many instances is extremely low, something that few physicians have previously experienced. Because the rates are not high, doctors have been calling them normal. But the very low levels are themselves abnormal, seen in only a handful of rare illnesses. In patients with CFIDS, it is common to see a sed rate of 0, 1, or 2 mm per hour. That is, the blood cells in the tube do not separate from the surrounding fluids and settle to the bottom at the normal rate. While by itself not diagnostic, the sed rate is a simple and inexpensive test, and should be part of the basic laboratory workup.

Routine Chemistries

Most laboratories have a battery of routine chemistries to detect common abnormalities in liver function, kidney function, bone abnormalities, and a variety of other disorders. Routine chemistries are screening tests that can detect disease states such as diabetes mellitus, hepatitis, and kidney failure. In CFIDS these tests are normal, except that up to 25 percent of patients may have minimal elevation of liver functions (Komaroff 88). However, this elevation of liver enzymes is usually so mild that concern is not raised. It is certainly not as high as in infectious hepatitis. Serious abnormalities on the chemistries should raise suspicion that some process other than CFIDS is causing the symptoms.

Thyroid Screen

Most chemistry panels will also test the thyroid hormones. This is important in CFIDS because thyroid abnormalities may cause fatigue and need to be excluded. In general the thyroid hormone levels are normal. However, in our office we have seen several patients who initially had normal thyroid testing but have developed thyroid abnormalities after having had CFIDS for several years. Therefore, we repeat the thyroid hormone levels at least on a yearly basis in patients with CFIDS. Any patient with abnormal thyroid hormone levels should be treated in the standard manner.

Thyroid Antibodies

These tests measure antibodies against thyroid tissue and are present in an illness known as thyroiditis. Patients with CFIDS occasionally have thyroid autoantibodies, which may present special problems in management. If thyroid function is impaired, it should be treated.

HIV Antibody

The HIV antibody is the standard test for AIDS, and any patient who received a blood transfusion in the early 1980s or who has any of the risk factors for AIDS should be screened. As unpleasant as it sounds, the symptoms of early AIDS are similar to CFIDS. The HIV test also serves to relieve anxiety, as many patients fear that somehow they may have caught AIDS. Having a negative test eliminates this fear.

Rheumatoid Factor (RF)

Most patients with CFIDS have joint pain, and it is necessary to exclude rheumatoid arthritis, an illness that also causes prominent fatigue. The vast majority of patients with CFIDS have a negative RF, which, in combination with a low sed rate, can eliminate rheumatoid arthritis as a possibility. On occasion a CFIDS patient may have a low level of rheumatoid factor.

Antinuclear Antibody (ANA)

This test measures antibodies directed against nuclear material of human cells and is found in high concentrations in patients with lupus erythematosis, another illness with joint pain and fatigue. Up to 20 percent of patients with CFIDS have low levels of ANA (Komaroff 88). However, instead of the steady elevation seen in lupus, the ANA seen in CFIDS is at low levels and variable. The fluctuating ANA, in combination with low sed rate and negative anti-DNA antibodies, excludes lupus as a diagnostic possibility.

Lyme Disease Antibodies

Lyme disease is caused by an infection with the bacteria Borrelia burgdorfi, usually transmitted by tick bite, and in the chronic form it may have many symptoms in common with CFIDS. Therefore, it is useful to measure the antibodies to this bacteria, particularly for patients living in areas where Lyme disease is common.

Chest X Ray

The chest X ray is normal in CFIDS and is valuable as a general screening tool for other infections, malignancies, and sarcoidosis. An abnormal chest X ray would suggest a diagnosis other than CFIDS. Sarcoidosis, an unusual disease featuring fatigue, is particularly interesting because it shares many symptoms and abnormal immunology with CFIDS.

Urinalysis

Another routine screening test, the urinalysis is usually normal in CFIDS, and a normal test eliminates several other diseases that may cause fatigue. Although symptoms of urgency and burning may be present in the patient with CFIDS, urine cultures are normal, which excludes infection of the urinary tract.

More Invasive Tests

The preceding tests are a reasonable basic diagnostic workup for patients with CFIDS and can exclude many other illnesses that prominently feature fatigue as a symptom. Further testing depends on the severity of illness, the pattern of symptoms, and the clinical judgment of the physician. If a patient is very ill, further exclusionary testing is certainly warranted; it would be a mistake to attribute all fatigue to CFIDS. The tests mentioned below are the more invasive tests and are used to eliminate other serious illnesses. Whether or not these tests are ordered is completely dependent on the clinical judgment of the physician.

Lumbar Puncture

A physician who is concerned about the possibility of multiple sclerosis or other diseases of the brain may suggest a lumbar puncture, otherwise known as a spinal tap. Although the tests for MS are negative in CFIDS, occasional patients may have slight unexplained elevations in the protein or cell count of the spinal fluid (Komaroff 88; Warner 89). If a lumbar puncture is undertaken, a careful reading of the spinal fluid pressure should be obtained, because this may help in treating the frequent headaches. Spinal taps for patients with CFIDS are difficult but are usually not dangerous. It is likely that the temporary change in spinal fluid pressure caused by the tap will precipitate a relapse in symptoms. However, if a spinal tap is indicated on clinical grounds, it should be done.

Upper and Lower GI Series

Abdominal complaints are common in CFIDS, and these X rays are frequently ordered to look for diseases such as duodenal or gastric ulcer, Crohn's disease, or ulcerative colitis. In addition, bowel endoscopy (peering into the bowel through a small tube) is used to diagnose certain diseases. In CFIDS, all these tests are normal, and no obvious cause for the bowel symptoms will be found. However, in any patient with severe bowel symptoms, these tests should be done, for the treatment of these other illnesses is quite different from CFIDS. It is particularly important to have these studies if blood is present in the stool, a rare finding in CFIDS.

Liver and Spleen Scan

This test is sometimes ordered because of pain in the area of the liver and spleen. A radionucleide is injected into the arm and collected by the liver and spleen. Measurements taken are able to show the size and shape of both the liver and spleen. Some diseases, including cancer, are noted by abnormalities in these tests. Aside from an occasional reading of mild enlargement, it is negative in CFIDS.

Bone Marrow Aspirate

In this uncomfortable test the cells of the bone marrow are removed and examined for different illnesses. This may be ordered when the physician is concerned about malignancy, particularly leukemia. I rarely perform this diagnostic test, but if indications are present, the test should be done. In CFIDS the results of standard staining of bone marrow cells are normal.

Lymph Node Biopsy

In many CFIDS patients the lymph nodes are tender, and 10 percent of patients may have some enlargement. Physicians may be concerned with the possibility of diseases such as tuberculosis, sarcoidosis, lymphoma, or Hodgkin's disease and may suggest a biopsy of the lymph node. Many of my patients had such a biopsy to rule out these illnesses. In patients with CFIDS who have a lymph node biopsy, the results show nonspecific findings known as reactive hyperplasia, which implies immune system activation, a topic to be discussed later. However, in general, anyone who has persistent enlargement of the lymph nodes (not necessarily discomfort in the lymph nodes) should have a biopsy.

CT Scan of the Brain

Because of severe headaches, many patients have a CT scan of the brain, a computerized set of X rays, to rule out brain tumor and other brain diseases. The test, usually normal in CFIDS, should be done on any patient with severe headache and neurologic symptoms. As will be mentioned in the chapter on research tests, an MRI scan can also rule out other pathological conditions and may add information on CFIDS. However, the MRI is a more expensive test than the CT scan.

Other Tests

There are numerous other illnesses that a physician may want to exclude based on the specific pattern of symptoms. These include infections with toxoplasmosis, cytomegalovirus, syphilis, tuberculosis, and others. If a patient's symptoms suggest any other specific illnesses, testing for those illnesses should be done.

Conclusion

Patients with CFIDS often undergo numerous laboratory tests, and to their dismay, the tests are negative. These patients should not be dismayed by lack of tumors, multiple sclerosis, and degenerative diseases of the brain—illnesses that are far worse than CFIDS. This is not to imply that CFIDS is a pleasant illness, but it is better than some.

The difficulty for patients with CFIDS is that when all the diagnostic tests come out negative, they are told that nothing is wrong and are dismissed by the physician. The problem is not the normal laboratory tests, it is the physician's lack of familiarity with CFIDS. But the lack of a diagnosis distresses the patients, because they understand and experience that something is wrong. However, with the growing understanding and acceptance of the specific symptom pattern of this illness, the problem that has been so devastating in the past is resolving. I hope that I will not be called a naive optimist several years from now.

CHAPTER 6

The Immunology of CFIDS

The name CFIDS was suggested by Dr. Seymour Grufferman, at a conference in 1987, to distinguish the illness from the common, garden-variety fatigue with which it is so often confused. But while immune system dysfunction is present, the majority of immunologic abnormalities in patients with CFIDS are subtle. Numerous abnormalities have been observed over the past several years, yet, like the pattern of symptoms, the pattern of immune abnormalities has defied simple classification. An understanding of the immunology of this illness is important in understanding why CFIDS is unique. This chapter reviews these immune system abnormalities and the tests that are used to discover them.

Some physicians have said that these abnormalities are trivial and represent only variations of the immune abnormalities of depression. Yet I do not believe they are trivial, and, as previously discussed, there is mounting evidence that suggests they are quite different from those found in depression. But, as with the routine laboratory tests reviewed in the preceding chapter, immunologic studies are not diagnostic. They are expensive and difficult to perform, and do not necessarily need to be performed on patients suspected of having CFIDS. It is rare that the results of immunologic studies have altered the clinical diagnosis of CFIDS.

As with many illnesses affecting the immune system, the abnormalities are not confined to one discrete area, or arm, of the immune system, but cross boundary lines. In CFIDS, some tests imply that the immune system is unable to mount a strong defensive response, although adequate enough to handle most regular infections. Other tests imply that the immune system is overactive, as if it were running wild. It is this irregular pattern of over- and underfunctioning that generated the term *immune dysfunction*. In our discussion we will look at the immune dysfunction of CFIDS by examining both of these areas. Although immune system underactivity, or suppression, is addressed first, it is likely to be the less important of the two.

*I*mmune System Suppression

Immune suppression generally means a poor immune response. It implies that the responses are underactive or dampened. It is as though sand had been thrown into the immune system machinery and the normal aggressive immunologic response has slowed down in several areas. In CFIDS, an underactive immune response is seen in discrete areas, but probably causes little functional harm or damage. Several different tests may show the poor response, but it is likely that very few of the symptoms of CFIDS are actually due to these abnormalities. Furthermore, they may not occur in every patient, may be mild, and may be intermittent. However, these abnormalities are clearly present more frequently than would be expected in healthy people or in people with primary emotional illness.

Viral Reactivation

As will be discussed in chapter seven, early studies in this country were focused around elevated antibody levels to several viral agents, including the Epstein-Barr virus (EBV), human herpes virus 6 (HHV-6), and other herpes group viruses. It now appears that these viral agents circulate in larger amounts in patients with CFIDS not because they are causing the illness but because the immune system is suppressed, allowing them more freedom to replicate. One way to conceptualize this is that the immune system is ignoring the tedious daily chore of suppressing latent viruses, perhaps because of illness, perhaps because it is occupied with other matters. However, these viruses do not replicate to the extent that they pose a serious risk to the patient's health. Measuring the antibody levels of these viruses may indirectly reflect the degree of immune system suppression. These agents do not cause CFIDS, but are innocent bystanders that, because of immune suppression, have been dragged into the complex picture of this illness.

Other Agent Reactivation

For years some clinicians and researchers have been maintaining that the common yeast candida is the cause of symptoms associated with CFIDS. *Chronic Fatigue and the Yeast Connection* by Dr. William Crook describes this in detail, and it has been a common experience of many clinicians that patients with CFIDS have an unnatural overgrowth of the yeast candida. In my own experience at least 20 percent of patients have some history of oral candidiasis. Dr. Carol Jessop has reported that over 80 percent of CFIDS patients will have evidence of candida by staining scraping taken from the mouth.

Some reports have suggested higher levels of antibodies to candida than should be expected in the general population, but the medical literature has not borne this out (Renfro 89). Like the Epstein-Barr virus, candida is ubiquitous, and is seen in AIDS and other diseases known to have immunosuppression. I believe the presence of candidiasis is a sign of poor immune functioning, not just infection with yeast.

Decreased Antibody Levels

While specific antibodies may be elevated to certain common viral and nonviral agents, overall level of antibody (immunoglobulin) may be low (Straus 88; Komaroff 88; DuBois 84; Lloyd 89). Moreover, if the types of antibody are subdivided, two subclasses of immunoglobulin, IgG1 and IgG3, may be low in patients with CFIDS (Komaroff 88; Lloyd 89; Peterson 90). This subclass is felt to be responsible for keeping viral infections in check.

Traditionally, it has been low levels of antibody that have acted as the primary marker for immune incompetence or immune suppression, the inability to generate antibodies to fight off infections. There are a great many conditions in which the body's ability to make antibodies is impaired, and this area has been studied extensively. In CFIDS the degree of these irregularities is relatively minor and does not present a threat of overwhelming infection. Patients with CFIDS usually do not get serious secondary infections such as pneumonia or abscesses. But in one interesting study, pneumoccal vaccine was given to patients with CFIDS, and it was noted that their ability to make pneumoccal antibody was impaired (Gupta 91).

Measuring immunoglobulins may be helpful in the overall evaluation for CFIDS, but they alone do not make the diagnosis.

Decreased Cell-Mediated Immunity

Abnormalities have been demonstrated in the area of delayed hypersensitivity (Murdoch 88; Lloyd 92). In these studies the degree of skin inflammation to common antigens is measured and then compared to normal reactivity. The normal response should be vigorous, with redness and swelling, but in CFIDS and several other disease states, little or no response is seen. The arm of the immune system controlling this response, cell-mediated immunity, is independent of the overall level of antibodies. In the studies published so far, only rough screening tests of cell-mediated immunity have been done, and more detailed studies to understand the meaning of these results are needed. However, like the antibody levels, decreased cell-mediated immunity is not specific for CFIDS. Yet the finding may add to the overall picture of immune dysfunction. Compared to other tests of immune function, it is inexpensive and one of the most useful.

Low Natural Killer Cell Number and Function

Natural killer cells, despite the ominous name, are normal lymphocytes that participate in several important aspects of the immune response. As early as 1985 abnormalities in both the number and the functioning of natural killer cells in CFIDS have been noted (Behan 85; Kibler 85; Franco 87; Salvato 88; Grufferman 88; Caligiuri 87; Klimas 90; Gupta 91). The evaluation of natural killer cell number and function is an important part of the diagnostic evaluation in patients with serious illness. Unfortunately, the test is difficult and expensive, and must be done by experts within a short time after the blood is drawn. Testing through commercial laboratories can evaluate the number of natural killer cells but not their function. In general, these tests should be reserved for research studies only.

Decreased Mitogen Responses

Numerous chemicals called mitogens are known to stimulate immunity. Lymphocytes replicate when exposed to mitogens, and it has been noticed that this response is blunted in CFIDS (Salvato 88; Lloyd 89). Like the natural killer cell studies, they are complicated, expensive, and difficult to perform and interpret. The degree of suppressed mitogen response is variable, and not all patients show these responses. The decreased mitogen activity may be due to exhaustion of the immune response.

Immune System Activation

Immune suppression can be thought of as the immune system paying little attention to certain functions because it is preoccupied somewhere else. The immune system may be compared to a busy office, and when a crisis arises in one area, the office becomes preoccupied with that crisis so that the paperwork and other routine matters are ignored.

A reflection of this preoccupation is seen in tests that measure immune system activation, or up-regulation, tests showing an overactive immune response. The immune system is functioning excessively in these areas, without a clear explanation as to why. As will be discussed later, the up-regulation may be an attempt to respond to Agent X, the theoretical cause of CFIDS.

Presence of Allergies

Multiple allergies are perhaps the most obvious sign of immune system overreaction. Patients with CFIDS frequently have a past history of allergies, implying that their immune response is genetically primed for a vigorous response. Other patients with CFIDS develop allergic symptoms after the onset of their illness. CFIDS patients have a hair trigger for allergies.

Allergies can be thought of as an exaggerated reaction of the immune system to harmless allergens, such as pollen and dust. In our model, the overreaction is another sign that in CFIDS the immune system is desperately trying to attack or suppress something. The immune system is like an angry man, fighting against enemies at work, carrying this anger home, and yelling at the harmless play of the children. The immune system will react against everything—pollen, dust, foods, odors, chemicals—even if these environmental factors are not causing damage.

Autoantibody Production

Autoimmunity is an abnormality of the immune system in which the body produces antibodies that react against itself. One current theory is that the immune system produces antibodies against viral or bacterial invaders and these antibodies cross-react with normal body tissues. This is likely when there is a structural similarity between the virus being attacked and a specific body tissue. An example of this type of autoantibody is present in rheumatic fever, where an antibody that reacts with heart tissue is produced.

A second possibility is that the immune system makes antibodies to normal tissue because of some error in interpretation of what is normal and what is an invader. Autoimmunity has been studied for years, and many diseases—such as lupus erythematosis, multiple sclerosis, and hypothyroidism—are felt to be caused by autoimmune phenomena. Autoimmunity is a process, however, and not a disease in itself. The diseases caused are the result of this process being directed against a specific target organ over a period of time. In thyroiditis, for example, the body makes antibodies that react with thyroid tissue, causing thyroid inflammation and gradual destruction. The autoimmune process in this case is directed against thyroid tissue and results in decreased ability of the thyroid to produce thyroid hormone.

The presence of autoimmunity in CFIDS has long been recognized. Up to 20 percent of patients have low levels of the antinuclear antibody, the test that usually detects lupus erythematosis (Salit 85; Straus 88; Murdoch 87). This antibody, the ANA, is directed against the cell's nuclear material and is generally present in quantities much less than what would be expected in lupus. CFIDS has been confused with lupus, and sometimes even called antibody negative lupus, but more specific tests for lupus are negative.

Ten percent of patients with CFIDS have low levels of rheumatoid factor, associated with rheumatoid arthritis. Again it is in lower concentrations than found in true rheumatoid arthritis. Up to 20 percent of CFIDS patients have antibody directed against smooth muscle, and 10 percent have antibodies to gastric parietal cells. Twenty percent have antibodies directed against thyroid tissue. This formation of antibodies against several tissue types demonstrates a general tendency in CFIDS for the formation of autoantibody. CFIDS is not caused by one specific type of autoantibody. It is intriguing to speculate, however, on possible relationships between CFIDS and other autoimmune diseases such as lupus or rheumatoid arthritis.

Other illnesses are known to have an increased incidence of autoimmune phenomena, AIDS being among them. Therefore, the process is again not specific. It can be thought of as a sign of hyperimmunity or exaggerated immune response, where the body, perhaps in a reckless attempt to fight some Agent X, is responding by attacking even itself.

Increased T8 Lymphocytes

Lymphocytes are one of the primary components of blood cells involved in the immune response, and it has been noted in some studies that the proportion of lymphocytes present in patients with CFIDS is altered. One type of lymphocyte, the T8 (sometimes called the T suppressor lymphocyte) may be present in increased percentages. This change in percentage affects the ratio of lymphocytes, measured as the T4/T8 ratio, a test often performed on patients with CFIDS. Patients with severe CFIDS may have elevations in this ratio, usually due to elevations in the T8 lymphocyte, although this is variable. There have been many studies on this question, and the results have been conflicting (Behan 85; Komaroff 88; Salvato 88; Klimas 90; Landay 91; Buchwald 92). Again, even if there is an elevation in the ratio of T suppressor lymphocytes, it is not specific for CFIDS.

Recently an illness characterized by low numbers of T helper lymphocytes (T4) has been described in patients who were suspected of having the HIV virus but in fact did not. Some patients with typical CFIDS will be found to have low T4 counts. It is likely that severe CFIDS and what has been called antibody-negative AIDS may prove to be the same illness.

Circulating Immune Complexes

Immune complexes circulating in the bloodstream can be detected in many illnesses. These antibodies are bound to protein and may be detected by several techniques. It is another nonspecific finding in CFIDS, one of the first noted, and probably reflects an increased activity of antibody reactions in general (Straus 85; Straus 88).

Interleukin-2 System Activation

Interleukins are cytokines, messenger chemicals normally produced by several different types of cells. Nearly twenty different interleukins have been identified so far, and the list is growing. Interleukin-2 (IL-2) was discovered in 1978 and originally was known as T-cell growth factor because, when added to lymphocyte cell cultures, it would cause T-cells to divide rapidly and grow in cell culture. It has been studied extensively and can be measured by a blood test.

In an attempt to find a marker for the immune system activation of CFIDS, Dr. Paul Cheney and I undertook a study of more than one hundred adult patients, and found elevated circulating levels of Interleukin-2 (Cheney 89). Patients in New York had the same pattern of elevation as patients in North Carolina, implying that this elevation was a function of the illness and not of a specific trigger factor. The test used in this study was an augmented interleukin-2 assay and is not readily found in commercial laboratories.

However, some patients, frequently the more ill, had normal levels of IL-2; and some of these patients had elevated interleukin-2 soluble receptor. In looking at the IL-2 system, composed of both IL-2 and the IL-2 soluble receptor, over 70 percent of patients with CFIDS had abnormal results (unpublished observation). Furthermore, there appeared to be a pattern of abnormality that was dependent on the degree or stage of illness. However, early hopes that IL-2 or its receptor might prove to be a marker for the illness have proven disappointing, as this finding has not been confirmed.

The presence of IL-2 and its receptor means that the immune system is activated—it is actively trying to do something. The immune system does not become activated by itself; there are too many checks and balances. It is activated because something activates it, presumably our Agent X, and not because of boredom, a yuppie lifestyle, or simple depression. Whatever activates the immune system is important enough for the body to risk serious overreaction, and the consequent problems, to try to fight it. The presence of IL-2 and/or its receptor means that something very serious is going on.

Published studies have shown that when isolated cells are stimulated, lower than expected amounts of IL-2 are produced (Kibler 85), and that adding IL-2 to natural killer cells does not stimulate them to the normal degree (Caligiuri 87). Both of these findings can be explained by exhaustion caused by chronic activation of the IL-2 system. Other interleukins, such as IL-1, may also be involved in CFIDS (Cotton 91; Linde 92). Further studies of these intriguing possibilities are under way.

Increased Interferon Production

A substance in the immune system that prevents replication of viruses was recognized over twenty years ago. This chemical "interfered" with viral replication and was called interferon. We now know of three general types of interferon, named alpha, beta, and gamma. Broadly speaking, the detection of interferon implies the presence of viral infection.

In CFIDS, the presence of interferon in increased amounts has long been suspected. Numerous investigators have noticed the presence of an enzyme system thought to be a marker for interferon (Straus 85; Ho-Yen 88; Straus 88). However, direct detection of interferon has been more difficult. There are two methods to measure interferon: direct measurement of the chemical through a test called IFA, and measurement of the biologic activity caused by interferon. The former test reveals that up to 20 percent of patients have alpha interferon (unpublished observation); the latter test shows a lower percentage positive (Kibler 85; Straus 85; Ho-Yen 88). This may imply either that the interferon present is not functioning normally or that the IFA test is picking up something that is not alpha interferon. On the other hand, the presence of the enzyme system implies localized production of interferon, which the blood test might not measure. In one study, alpha interferon was found to be elevated in spinal fluid of patients with CFIDS (Lloyd, Hickie et al. 91). Much more research in this area is needed.

The presence of an activated interferon cellular enzyme system implies that the interferon system is switched on. This is another reflection of immunologic activation or up-regulation. It again implies that the immune system is activated and searching for something to attack, presumably a virus. While the results of interferon levels are intriguing, not enough patients are positive for the test to be useful as a standard diagnostic marker.

Conclusion

Numerous immunologic abnormalities have been seen on specific testing of patients with CFIDS. Some tests imply a poorly functioning immune system, some an overactive immunity. This bizarre pattern has been difficult to confirm because of test variability among laboratories and the expense of scientific studies. No single test of immune functioning is diagnostic. Like the symptoms, the pattern of immunologic results is more important than the specific results of a single test. Whether the pattern of abnormalities will help to make the diagnosis in the future remains to be seen, but preliminary findings have been encouraging.

It is difficult to know why this pattern of immune dysfunction exists without knowing the cause of CFIDS. But the pattern is not random. It suggests an alteration or disruption in function consisting of simultaneous overresponse in some directions and neglect in others. One persisting hypothesis is that the abnormal response is directed toward a difficult-to-find invading organism, one able to interfere with basic immunologic mechanisms.

Extensive immunologic testing is usually not necessary in patients with CFIDS, and because of the expense, I perform these tests only on those patients who are very ill. In general, the more severely ill a patient, the more likely that tests of immune functioning will be outside the normal range. More accurate assessment of the degree of these abnormalities, as well as standardization of laboratory testing, is necessary before it can become routine. What is certain, however, is that CFIDS patients do demonstrate abnormal immunity, measurable on numerous laboratory tests.

In a recent paper, Dr. Nancy Klimas stated, "CFS is a form of acquired immunodeficiency" (Klimas 90). This one study alone makes the argument as to whether CFIDS is a real illness somewhat absurd.

CHAPTER 7

Epstein-Barr Virus

*A*s we have seen, elevations have been found in antibody levels to certain viruses. The first descriptions of the symptom complex we now call CFIDS in the United States were associated with unusual antibody levels to the Epstein-Barr virus (EBV), which is the usual cause of infectious mononucleosis. In 1982 Tobi and his coworkers described an illness linked to elevations in EBV antibodies. In 1985 Jones and Straus wrote papers describing this illness in more detail.

Then came the outbreak of Incline Village, Nevada, described in 1985 by Dr. Daniel Peterson and Dr. Paul Cheney—a milestone in the study of CFIDS. It is possible that many physicians had seen patients with the complex symptoms of CFIDS without recognizing it as a discrete syndrome because it had not been clearly defined. With the Incline Village outbreak, the two physicians were able to define the clinical syndrome in an epidemic population and link it to a possible biologic marker, elevated antibody levels to the Epstein-Barr virus. The ensuing publicity and the label of "yuppie flu," although demeaning, focused attention on the subsequent controversy of whether there was a specific illness present or merely mass hysteria. This, combined with the Epstein-Barr virus marker, allowed attention to be drawn to CFIDS in a way that had not occurred previously in this country. The confusion concerning the link between the two still lingers and therefore merits a closer examination.

The Epstein-Barr virus was discovered by three researchers, Epstein, Achong, and Barr, in 1964 while studying a lymphoma common in Africa, the Burkitt's lymphoma. It was subsequently noted to be the most common cause of infectious mononucleosis, and eloquent studies on the natural history and pathogenesis of this virus have been conducted.

It is now known that almost all adults, up to 95 percent, have had an infection with the Epstein-Barr virus at some time during their life. If this infection took place in early childhood, it may not have been recognized or may have been a mild flulike illness. If the infection was severe, or occurred for the first time during adolescence, infectious mononucleosis was diagnosed. Although not everyone develops infectious mono, in those who do it is usually the result of primary infection with EBV.

EBV belongs to the herpes virus family and, like other herpes viruses, can never be totally eradicated. The virus remains present in the body, and can be cultured from the saliva and other fluids from time to time. A healthy immune system can control replication and keep the virus in a latent state so that ongoing symptoms do not occur.

However, EBV can cause severe and sometimes fatal infections if the body's immune mechanism is not functioning properly. Severe "chronic Epstein-Barr virus" infection (CEBV) is known to occur with several inherited immune deficiencies, and can occur with immune system suppression due to bone marrow failure or with drugs used to treat malignancies. CEBV has been studied since the discovery of EBV and is not new.

The initial hypothesis concerning the Epstein-Barr virus and CFIDS in North America was simple enough: that this virus was somehow causing the illness. Perhaps, for whatever reason, the virus or another strain of EBV was out of control and therefore causing a "chronic mononucleosis," a term that arose because of the nature of the symptoms and the elevated antibody levels. This name, and the term chronic Epstein-Barr virus infection (CEBV), became the first terms for CFIDS used in this country, and the publicity around the illness centered on the role of the Epstein-Barr virus as the cause of CFIDS.

The outbreak in Incline Village and other areas was not like the known cases of CEBV. First, CEBV is due to very severe immune deficiency and is unlikely to occur in epidemics. Second, the level of EBV antibody elevation seen is not as great as in true CEBV. Third, and most important, patients with this new problem did not have the severe, life-threatening course that is seen in true chronic EBV infections. I remember a patient-oriented conference on CFIDS during which one speaker discussed true CEBV. When he mentioned the mortality rate of over 50 percent, the audience groaned. True chronic Epstein-Barr virus infection and CFIDS are not the same disease.

The Debate over EBV Antibodies

One of the most important mechanisms that keep EBV in a controlled state is the presence of several different antibodies. If a person has never been exposed to the Epstein-Barr virus, none of these antibodies are found in the blood. However, because up to 95 percent of adults have had an infection with this virus, the antibodies are present in "normal" quantities, implying that the virus is under control. The three patterns of EBV antibodies are (1) no antibodies present, implying that there has never been an infection; (2) high levels of antibodies, implying an acute infection; and (3) low levels of antibodies, implying an infection at some time in the past.

In CFIDS roughly one-third of the adults have unusual and abnormal levels. These levels are unusual because they suggest both past infection and recent infection. This pattern has been called chronic infection or reactivation pattern because it could be explained if an individual had a primary EBV infection years previously and is now fighting the virus again. That is, there had been a previous infection but there is also an active current infection. Thus another name for patients with this pattern was "chronic active EBV infection." The remaining two-thirds of patients with CFIDS had antibody levels that are no different from the general population.

Although the involvement of the Epstein-Barr virus was superficially appealing, virologists and other scientists pointed out numerous holes in the hypothesis. First, only one-third of patients had unusual levels of EBV antibodies, and the severity of symptoms did not correlate with the degree of abnormality in antibody levels. Furthermore, the pattern of antibody levels was unlike true chronic EBV infection. Did this mean that one-third had a chronic Epstein-Barr virus infection and the remaining two thirds had some other disease? This didn't make sense because an outbreak or epidemic should have a single cause.

Several studies on patients with CFIDS have not shown elevated EBV antibody levels. One study was among children in an epidemic in Lyndonville, New York, in 1985. Nearly all adults have antibodies to EBV in their blood, but children are less likely to have been exposed. In the Lyndonville cluster, the illness occurred in three or more children in some families. In studying these children, it was clear that they all had the same illness, judging by the symptoms, clinical course, and physical findings, and because they became ill at the same time. But measuring the antibodies to the Epstein-Barr virus, 25 percent had no antibodies at all (meaning they had never been exposed to the virus), 50 percent had "normal" levels of antibodies (implying some past infection), and 25 percent had high levels (implying reactivation). The absence of antibodies in 25 percent is expected in children of this age group, and the obvious conclusion was that CFIDS could occur independently of a past Epstein-Barr virus. Because the symptoms were not related to antibody levels, the symptoms could not be caused by the Epstein-Barr virus. Thus CFIDS could not be "caused" by the Epstein-Barr virus in this group of children (Bell 88).

Another criticism was that elevated antibody levels to the Epstein-Barr virus are seen in other conditions. It is possible that fifty separate illnesses ranging from rheumatoid arthritis to malignancy, demonstrate elevated EBV antibody levels. Therefore, even if the levels are elevated, they are not specific for CFIDS. Even in some normal conditions, such as old age and pregnancy, the antibody control of the Epstein-Barr virus is not entirely effective and the levels fluctuate. Thus doubt arose in numerous areas simultaneously, and what at first seemed to be a marker for this illness was now being dismissed as meaningless. The research on CFIDS in America seemed to be back at stage zero.

Although many physicians completely dismissed the findings concerning the Epstein-Barr virus, others did not. Several things have become apparent, among them that some patients with CFIDS have a reactivation of latent infection with the Epstein-Barr virus. Also, EBV may be important in triggering the illness in some patients.

Evidence now exists showing altered immunity in CFIDS, and this defect in immunity allows for reactivation of viruses in several classes. Other studies have found elevated antibody levels to other herpes viruses and enteroviruses. Elevated antibody levels to different viruses do not imply separate illnesses; they imply that the primary problem is the immune dysfunction that permits them. What causes the immune dysfunction is the central problem in CFIDS. The emphasis in research is shifting from the details of specific viruses to the cause of the immune dysfunction.

The Concept of EBV as a Trigger Infection

Many patients with CFIDS first became ill with an episode of infectious mononucleosis. This by itself seemed to implicate the Epstein-Barr virus as the causative agent. However, two explanations can exonerate EBV. The first question to ask is: Was it EBV that caused the infectious mononucleosis? Not necessarily.

Infectious mononucleosis can be caused by numerous agents, such as toxoplasmosis, cytomegalovirus, and HHV-6. Many times the diagnosis of EBV-induced infectious mononucleosis is merely an assumption, because without the very specific EBV antibodies, the diagnosis is not certain. Therefore, when a patient states that the CFIDS began with infectious mononucleosis, we are still not certain that it is the Epstein-Barr virus unless EBV antibodies were measured. Yet most researchers have indeed seen patients whose CFIDS began with verified EBV infection.

This raises the possibility that EBV infection may trigger CFIDS, while not necessarily causing it. As mentioned in chapter two, other agents may trigger CFIDS as well. Most researchers have heard patients say that their illness began after a period of intense stress, measles vaccine, or toxic fume exposure. If this is true, why does CFIDS occur after an event that should cause no long-term illness? Is it a coincidence that several different agents cause the same constellation of symptoms, or is some as yet unidentified cause (our Agent X) merely waiting to be triggered?

Another factor should be added. As discussed previously, at least 25 percent of patients do not have an acute onset of their symptoms but gradually develop symptoms over long periods of time. Moreover, many of those with an acute onset had mild symptoms prior to developing CFIDS, the "vulnerable period." Therefore, it is possible that a trigger agent precipitates a problem that would otherwise have presented in a more subtle, and perhaps milder, form.

Conclusion

The research on the Epstein-Barr virus and numerous other agents involved with CFIDS has been important in the understanding of the disease while at the same time creating confusion because of the complexity. CFIDS is like the story of the blind men feeling and describing an elephant; some describe the cylindrical trunk, some the ivory tusks, some the heavy round body. All are studying the same animal but are unable to communicate because they are experiencing something different.

In CFIDS we have some researchers devoting their time to the Epstein-Barr virus, some to human herpes 6, some to candida, and some to Coxsackie, all agents implicated in CFIDS at one time or another. There are probably numerous other agents where the phenomenon of elevated antibodies takes place. Even though it now appears that none of these agents is Agent X, each researcher is on the right track because behind the mystery of the reactivated agents lies the answer to what causes the immune dysfunction. It is a hope, shared by patients and researchers alike, that the cause is only one step behind these reactivated agents, not eight or nine.

CHAPTER 8

Research Testing

*P*hysicians skeptical of the existence of CFIDS as a discrete illness rightly demand a reproducible marker to show the existence of organic illness. Until this marker is found, arguments will persist about whether or not CFIDS is "real." Of course, this is not a new development in medicine. Multiple sclerosis was considered to be psychosomatic until the pathologic abnormalities of that illness were discovered.

Researchers convinced that CFIDS is a real illness have been searching for this biologic marker, one that will distinguish ill CFIDS patients from healthy people, and one that will reflect illness severity. Numerous abnormalities have been uncovered, but as of this writing none can stand alone as a marker for the illness. Some, perhaps many, of these exciting research findings may ultimately prove wrong, a dead end, although each finding is exciting and intriguing by itself. It may be many years before the present isolated puzzle pieces are joined into a meaningful and unified portrait. Until that time, these tests remain exploratory—much to the dismay of patients looking for definitive answers. None of these research tests can, by themselves, be used to establish a diagnosis.

For the most part, these tests should be performed only in rigorous research studies where their import may be accurately determined. But it is of some value to review these tests because they can also give us hints as to what may be underlying the illness. This chapter contains technical material, but is useful for those who wish to know what research is being done.

The Tests

Cognitive Testing

Patients with CFIDS consistently have cognitive symptoms, such as short-term memory loss, word-finding problems, and difficulty with attention. Tests of cognitive function are attempts at objectively measuring these deficits, but they are difficult and laborious to perform. They may be helpful in documenting the type of intellectual problems present and in evaluating the progression of the illness. It has been suggested that patients with severe symptoms have a CFIDS dementia. The testing should be carried out by specialists familiar with the patterns seen in CFIDS.

In an early study, abnormalities in frontal lobe functioning were noted, and the observation was made that the abnormalities were somewhat similar to those seen with the administration of the cytokine interferon (Jones 88a). This is of interest because of the possible role played by cytokines, to be discussed later.

Several other studies of cognitive function have been performed. In one, patients from the Incline Village outbreak demonstrated numerous deficits in cognitive performance, including difficulties with attention, verbal memory, problem solving, and sequencing ability. Simultaneous psychologic tests (MMPI) implied that the deficits were not due to malingering or primary psychological disturbance. Overall, the impairments were consistent with an "atypical organic brain syndrome" (Daugherty 91).

One study with similar findings noted that patients with CFIDS were slower and less accurate with working memory, and that the results were reliable over time (Smith 92). Another study goes so far as to state that the results of their testing "point to the presence of an organic, probably viral etiology for the neuropsychiatric abnormalities" (Riccio 92).

Do the cognitive deficits involve taking in information or in utilizing and processing information? One study attempting to address this question noted difficulties in response time, suggesting that there was no abnormality in perception and attention; the primary difficulty was in making responses (Scheffers 92).

Magnetic Resonance Imaging of the Brain (MRI Scan)

The MRI is a sensitive imaging test measuring magnetic resonance of bodily tissues, which has proven useful in diagnosing multiple sclerosis (MS). A longstanding controversy has surrounded its use in CFIDS. Some investigators maintain that scans in CFIDS patients show small abnormal areas, sometimes called "bright spots." The counterargument is that these spots can be found in normal people as well as in those ill with CFIDS (Buchwald 92; Daugherty 91; Cotton 91). However, it is clear that these spots are quite different from those found in MS, and do not progress to MS. Several investigators believe that the spots seen on MRI are an indicator of more severe neurologic problems, but this also has not yet been proven.

While the usefulness of the MRI scan has not been fully demonstrated, it is definitely helpful in ruling out MS as a cause for the neurologic symptoms. An MRI scan will also show brain abnormalities such as tumors, cysts, and pressure changes.

SPECT Scan

The SPECT scan, which measures brain blood flow, is an interesting new technology that may become very useful in the diagnosis and management of CFIDS. Illnesses that affect the blood flow to the brain will often have abnormal scans. Few reports have been published regarding its use in CFIDS, but some studies have shown abnormal brain blood flow (Goldstein 91; Costa 92; Douli 92; Troughton 92).

If these findings prove to be accurate, it supports an interesting hypothesis that has important therapeutic implications. Perhaps the symptoms of CFIDS are due to brain perfusion abnormalities similar to migraine? Perhaps, because not enough blood is reaching the midbrain, changes occur in midbrain function that do not cause permanent damage as would be seen in stroke or brain hemorrhage. If so, medications that stabilize blood vessels may be of value in treatment. SPECT scans are an exciting development, but they require more research.

Brain Mapping

Computerized brain-wave (EEG) technology, although very difficult to perform and interpret, is now becoming an accepted area of study. There have been no published papers on brain mapping in CFIDS, although several projects are under way. Difficulties in brain arousal causing poor attention should be demonstrated by this technology.

Sleep Studies

The study of sleep stages, although an imperfect science, may help in the evaluation of people suspected of having CFIDS. In a sleep study, a continuous brain wave is recorded during a night's sleep, and the progression of sleep stages is observed. Several illnesses with prominent fatigue, such as sleep apnea and narcolepsy, are unique in their sleep wave patterns. Some minor changes may be seen in sleep studies of patients with CFIDS, but large-scale trials are yet to be done (Krupp 91; Whelton 92).

Vestibular Studies

Tests of the balance mechanism in the middle ear and brain stem also offer an interesting avenue of research, and again, large definitive studies are yet to be done. Preliminary studies have suggested that some abnormalities in the brain stem itself may be related to the symptoms of dizziness and poor balance (Furman 91).

Abnormal Red Blood Cell Reology

One interesting avenue of research was opened by the publication of electron micrographs showing distorted shape of the red blood cells, which carry oxygen to the tissues throughout the body (Mukherjee 87; Simpson 86). If the blood cells are distorted in size and shape, they will not fit through the very small capillaries in the body tissues, including the brain. If the body is not receiving adequate oxygen, fatigue is one obvious result. Several researchers have noted tiny increases in bilirubin, which might be explained if the blood cells are of abnormal shape. However, there are no published reports.

It is an interesting hypothesis, one that has therapeutic implications. However, it has now been five years since this hypothesis was put forth and not much has come of it. Most researchers are not enthusiastic, yet published papers either confirming or denying the original study are lacking.

Angiotensin Converting Enzyme

In an isolated study, abnormalities of the angiotensin converting enzyme (usually found in blood vessels) were noted—abnormalities that, if confirmed, might help in the diagnosis of CFIDS (Lieberman 92). This enzyme is elevated in several conditions, most notably sarcoidosis and diseases of blood vessels. Sarcoidosis shares many symptoms of CFIDS.

Magnesium

In 1991, a paper was published demonstrating decreased red blood cell magnesium in thirty-one of thirty-two patients (Cox 91a & b). Moreover, treatment with magnesium not only returned the levels to normal but reduced symptoms. This exciting development unfortunately does not look as promising now as it did a year ago. Other studies have failed to confirm the original, and treatment with magnesium does not appear to be as dramatic as originally reported (Gantz 91; Clague 92; Durlach 92; Howard 92).

Adrenal Hormones

In an important 1991 paper, Demitrack and colleagues reported abnormal results in a study involving adrenal hormones. The results suggested a mild central adrenal insufficiency, implying that there was inadequate stimulus from the brain to the adrenal glands.

This report has several interesting implications. First, the response noted is quite different from that seen in primary depression, and helps to further separate the two illnesses. Second, it supports the concept of brain abnormalities in CFIDS, something that has long been suspected. Other related studies have shown an unusual brain response to excessive water loads (Behan, Goldberg and Mowbray 91). Unfortunately, these tests are difficult and cannot be routinely employed in the diagnosis of patients with suspected CFIDS. But further research in this area may lead to a greater understanding of the brain's role in this illness.

Skeletal Muscle Studies

One persisting controversy has been whether the weakness experienced by CFIDS patients is due to abnormalities within muscle or to perceptual difficulties within the brain. There have been numerous attempts to approach this problem, as it has important consequences for understanding the illness. If there are actual metabolic or structural problems within the muscle, then muscle biopsy would be of help in making the diagnosis. If the opposite is true, then it is the brain that is telling the CFIDS patient of weakness even though there is no disease within the muscle tissue itself.

Several studies have demonstrated some muscle atrophy and traces of viral infection by Coxsackie and other viruses (Archard 88; Lloyd 90; Warner 89; Behan, More and Behan 91). However, the muscle atrophy is not dramatic for the degree of symptoms, and the type of muscle fiber involved is the kind that can become weak with disuse. The finding of viral traces within the muscle tissue may be due to a persistence of viral infection affecting the muscle itself or to viral traces found in lymphocytes not fully separated from the muscle prior to testing.

Another approach is to examine the muscles themselves for their strength and durability. Early studies implied weakness that could be measured after exercise (Behan 85). More recent studies, however, show that despite the symptoms of weakness, the muscles seem to function as well in CFIDS patients as in healthy controls (Lloyd, Gandevia and Hales 91; Wood 91). "The feelings of weakness and fatigue experienced by the patients could not be explained by either physiological muscle fatigue or lack of effort"

(Rutherford 91). Electrical studies of the muscles have shown excessive jitter, the meaning of which is under dispute (Jamal 85; Behan 85).

Mitochondrial Abnormalities

The mitochondria are the part of cells that transform food into energy available for bodily functions. In any discussion of fatigue, mitochondrial abnormalities instantly become an attractive hypothesis. That so little work has been done on metabolic and mitochondrial studies in patients with CFIDS is surprising, especially since CFIDS exhibits a number of symptoms that are suggestive of mitochondrial disease: (a) onset of the illness by a viral infection; (b) worsening by stress or fasting; (c) unusual patterns of weight gain and loss; (d) occasional low blood sugar; and (e) familial component. Those studies that have been done display conflicting results.

Looking at the size and shape of mitochondria may reveal abnormalities in up to 75 percent of CFIDS patients, implying disease in the mitochondria themselves (Behan 85; Behan 91). But analysis of the metabolism has not revealed abnormalities in a small number of patients (Byrne 87; Byrne 88). However, these studies are extremely difficult to perform, and will not detect abnormalities unless all mitochondria are similarly affected. A more recent study has disclosed an abnormality that has great potential for future research. If correct, this study would imply that patients with CFIDS have either abnormal transport into the mitochondria, or mishandling of the foodstuffs in the process of being converted to energy (Kuratsone 92). It is an exciting lead that should be followed up with more studies.

Conclusion

Research on CFIDS is in its infancy, and two problems stand in the way of its development. The first and greatest obstacle is the the lack of research funding. It is only with the improved availability of funding that experts in such fields as sleep physiology, vestibular function, and mitochondrial metabolism will become interested and begin projects that will help answer the many questions. As CFIDS gets the recognition that has been lacking in years past, funding may improve.

The second obstacle is the difficulty in making a clinical diagnosis. What looks like CFIDS to one researcher may not to another. Therefore, in any study we must examine the criteria being used. The publication of the Centers for Disease Control criteria, although they certainly are not perfect, has helped overcome this problem to a great extent.

CHAPTER 9

The Measurement of Disability

*A*s we have learned, there is no lack of tests for the CFIDS patient. By the time every disease that CFIDS is often mistaken for has been ruled out, a patient might think he or she has had every exam ever invented by the medical community. Then at last the mysterious illness is diagnosed and acknowledged. Now what? More tests.

One of the most devastating effects of CFIDS is the profound disability it may produce. This is certainly not the case in all CFIDS patients; most patients recover either completely or to a good functional state. However, some are disabled, perhaps for the rest of their lives. For these patients, arriving at the appropriate diagnosis and management of disability is vital.

The medical assessment of CFIDS must include an accurate assessment of functional capacity, obtained by careful questioning and observation. Preferably, this assessment should be made over several visits with observations for consistency and the pattern of activity limitation seen in CFIDS. This assessment of functional capacity may be crucial to whether or not a disability claim is accepted.

As most patients are aware, there have been great obstacles in obtaining disability benefits, and CFIDS has only recently been recognized as a potentially disabling illness. We will not discuss the legal aspects of disability other than to state that, by law, the government provides financial support if a citizen is medically disabled. There are numerous publications that help patients gain these rights, generally available through patient support organizations. But many patients with milder CFIDS are able to work full time, and some who are quite sick recover completely. The problem facing the disability analyst is twofold: (1) how to make a diagnosis of CFIDS, and (2) which patient with CFIDS qualifies for disability.

Three separate factors are necessary for a patient to establish medical disability. The first, and perhaps the most important, is the opinion and diagnosis of the primary care physician as to the integrity and sincerity of the claimant. Second, documentation of the degree of disability over time, establishing both the prognosis and the seriousness of the physician in supporting a claim, is needed. And third, estimates of long-term prognosis, based on knowledge and experience with CFIDS, are necessary. Occasionally, documentation of abnormal neurocognitive or immunologic testing is helpful in supporting a claim.

The medical diagnosis has been covered in other parts of this book. Most patients with significant disability have abnormal immunological functioning, and documentation of these abnormalities may help to establish objective criteria useful to disability analysts. However, since the degree of abnormality noted on testing does not always represent the degree of disability, this has been a thorn. That is, some very disabled patients have relatively normal immune system testing, while some healthy people have a few minor abnormal immunological tests. Therefore, other measures are necessary in documenting the disability.

The Opinion of the Primary Care Physician

The patient's primary care physician is essential in this process. This physician usually knows the patient well, which is more important than expertise in CFIDS. The physician can describe in general terms the limitations caused by the illness. More important, an opinion may be given that the patient wants to work, and is honest, reliable, and industrious. On the other hand, the primary care physician might write that the patient is, and always has been, a bum. These opinions are, and should be, taken seriously by disability analysts. It is important for patients with CFIDS to maintain a close relationship with their primary care physician. He or she should be competent and caring, and be able to communicate an opinion of the claimant's honesty and desire to work.

That there is no single test that will measure disability is the crux of the problem. It would be very nice if a blood test could tell us that a patient could work hard physical labor six hours a day, five days a week, or could work a desk job without difficulty. But there is no completely objective measure of the degree of limitation imposed by CFIDS.

Different individuals have different levels of tolerance. This does not imply that some are faking it; it is not a wimp factor, but rather an acknowledgment that people are constructed differently. It is a factor that we need to understand and respect. I know a patient who would not apply for disability even on his deathbed because of what it represents for him. I also know a man who is so frightened by the illness and so devastated by the loss of previous abilities that he is applying for disability even though he is able to exert himself for four to five hours a day. Is one man better than the other? I don't think so, but they are different. I would support the disability claim of the first patient who won't apply and would not support the disability claim of the second who has applied. I believe that the second patient would, in the long run, be better off working full-time with some discomfort than on disability with the same discomfort. I think it would be better for his emotional state to be self-supporting, even though it is more difficult than it had previously been. Also, I think he may have a good chance of recovery.

In general I would support the disability claim of any patient whom I knew to be honest and clearly unable to work because of illness, and most physicians would apply the same criteria. Moreover, the activity limitation should be expected to continue for an extended period of time.

Cfids Disability Scale

One defining aspect of CFIDS is that with rest, many people feel relatively well, but symptoms flare up with exertion or activity. Some people with CFIDS will have three or fours hours a day when they feel relatively well, most commonly in the afternoon, the "activity window." It is during this time that they can shop or do activities outside the house with less difficulty. The disability in CFIDS is not the same as in cancer or multiple sclerosis where performance level is constant during the day and constant from day to day. Any good measure of the disability status in this illness needs to take these variables into account.

For the physician seeing a patient with CFIDS, it is useful to measure level of activity and ability to function with a simple instrument on every visit. This will document clinical improvement or its absence, note medication effects, and serve as a useful marker to the disability analyst. Moreover, it will help communicate that the disability and limitations claimed have been observed and taken seriously by the physician. Doctors dislike filling out tedious disability claims; their job is medical, not legal. But it is part of the physician's responsibility, and having good documentation over a period of time makes the process much easier.

One such instrument is the CFIDS Disability Scale, reproduced on the following page. The patient can fill it out while waiting for an office visit, and the physician may modify it with notes if necessary. It is a rating scale similar to other instruments but modified with a greater range in the area of disability seen in CFIDS. The attempt is to document as accurately as possible the severity of symptoms, the degree of activity impairment with both activity and rest, and the functional ability regarding full-time work. The principle behind this rating scale is that symptom severity is often related to exertion. This is bewildering to a disability analyst who says, "When you are sick, you're sick—*not* When you work, you're sick." The score assigned should be closest to the overall degree of limitation.

This disability rating scale has been developed in our office, and any physician wishing to use it may feel free to do so.

CFIDS Disability Scale

100: No symptoms at rest; no symptoms with exercise; normal overall activity level; able to work full-time without difficulty.

90: No symptoms at rest; mild symptoms with activity; normal overall activity level; able to work full-time without difficulty.

80: Mild symptoms at rest; symptoms worsened by exertion; minimal activity restriction noted for activities requiring exertion only; able to work full-time with difficulty in jobs requiring exertion.

70: Mild symptoms at rest; some daily activity limitation clearly noted. Overall functioning close to 90% of expected except for activities requiring exertion. Able to work full-time with difficulty.

60: Mild to moderate symptoms at rest; daily activity limitation clearly noted. Overall functioning 70%–90%. Unable to work full-time in jobs requiring physical labor, but able to work full-time in light activity if hours flexible.

50: Moderate symptoms at rest. Moderate to severe symptoms with exercise or activity; overall activity level reduced to 70% of expected. Unable to perform strenuous duties, but able to perform light duty or desk work 4–5 hours a day, but requires rest periods.

40: Moderate symptoms at rest. Moderate to severe symptoms with exercise or activity; overall activity level reduced to 50%–70% of expected. Not confined to house. Unable to perform strenuous duties; able to perform light duty or desk work 3–4 hours a day, but requires rest periods.

30: Moderate to severe symptoms at rest. Severe symptoms with any exercise; overall activity level reduced to 50% of expected. Usually confined to house. Unable to perform any strenuous tasks. Able to perform desk work 2–3 hours a day, but requires rest periods.

20: Moderate to severe symptoms at rest. Unable to perform strenuous activity; overall activity 30%–50% of expected. Unable to leave house except rarely; confined to bed most of day; unable to concentrate for more than 1 hour a day.

10: Severe symptoms at rest; bedridden the majority of the time. No travel outside of the house. Marked cognitive symptoms preventing concentration.

0: Severe symptoms on a continuous basis; bedridden constantly; unable to care for self.

One problem with this instrument is that it is new and has not been validated with large-scale scientific studies. It has the potential problem that a patient may be at a score of 50 in one area but a score of 30 in another, and in this case the physician may make the overall determination. A further problem is that it is subjective, and the scores may differ from physician to physician. Yet despite these limitations, this scale does give a general score that may be applicable to the type of disability seen in CFIDS.

*K*arnofsky Rating Scale

This simple rating method has been used for years in the evaluation of disability in disease states such as cancer and multiple sclerosis. Like almost all other methods, it is subjective and cannot be proven. But it is easy, useful, and remarkably consistent. The biggest obstacle with the Karnofsky Scale is that it is equally spread between healthy and dead. The majority of patients with CFIDS are grouped in a narrow band on this scale, so that both the sensitivity of this disability rating scale for CFIDS patients and the ability to show change over time are poor. However, the measure is useful because it is established and accepted as a measure of disability.

100: Normal with no complaints or evidence of disease.

90: Able to carry on normal activity but with minor signs of illness present.

80: Normal activity but requiring effort. Signs and symptoms of disease more prominent.

70: Able to care for self, but unable to work or carry on other normal activities.

60: Able to care for most needs, but requires occasional assistance.

50: Considerable assistance and frequent medical care required; some self-care possible.

40: Disabled, requiring special care and assistance.

30: Severely disabled; hospitalization required but death not imminent.

20: Extremely ill; supportive treatment and/or hospitalization required.

10: Imminent death.

0: Death.

Sickness Impact Profile

This copyrighted instrument, known as the SIP, measures the impact of an illness, any illness, on a person's life. Like the Karnofsky Scale, it is of value because it has been tested in many illnesses and is well known. The instrument is broken down into twelve separate areas: ambulation, mobility, body care/movement, social interaction, communication, alertness behavior, emotional behavior, sleep and rest, eating, work, home management, and recreational and pastime. Testing of this instrument in patients with CFIDS would be of value to determine if a specific disability pattern exists. It has the drawback of being subjective and because it is copyrighted, it requires written permission. However, it serves as an excellent instrument to evaluate function over time.

Kilocalorie Expenditure (Huang and Quinlan Method)

In 1988 Dr. Huang presented a method of measuring disability at a conference in Rome, Italy (Huang and Quinlan 89). The basis of the method is to calculate, based on calorie expenditure, the amount of disability present. If a patient keeps an accurate diary of daily activity, it is possible to calculate the kilocalorie expenditure for that day and compare it to established normals. This number can then be used as an objective measure of disability. In a patient with moderately severe CFIDS, the kilocalorie calculation shows a clear reduction in energy expenditure.

Although this method provides an objective measure of the disability, it is still subjective in that it requires an accurate history of the patient's daily activities. If a patient is dishonest in reporting daily activities, this method cannot detect it; therefore, the patient needs to record activity without exaggeration. Also, the calculation of energy expenditure is tedious for the physician.

Radial Plot of Symptoms

The radial plot of symptoms is a method attempting to coordinate the number of symptoms, their severity, and their pattern in a person with CFIDS. It is a modification of a method developed by Dr. Holmes and his New Zealand coworkers to evaluate abnormalities in laboratory evaluation, presented at the London Myalgic Encephalomyelitis conference in April 1990.

Like many other measures, it is a subjective evaluation of certain symptoms and their severity; in this respect it shares the drawbacks of other methods. However, this method requires a certain diagnostic pattern of symptoms to produce the high scores characteristically seen in CFIDS. Therefore, it is theoretically possible to differentiate CFIDS from other illnesses such as depression and somatization.

To date, this method has not been rigorously tested and therefore is still of unknown value in disability determination. However, it represents an interesting approach we have been developing in our office, and I present it as a follow-up tool for anyone wishing to pursue it further.

To calculate the radial plot, the patient fills out a questionnaire to determine the severity of each of twelve symptoms, with a range from 0 (no pain or problem) to 10 (very severe) for each symptom noted. The patient may complete this simple questionnaire prior to an appointment with a physician. The visual analog scales for each of the twelve symptoms are reproduced below.

Please mark an "x" next to the number that most closely represents the amount of pain or difficulty you have for each of the symptoms listed below. It should be representative of a typical day over the past month.

From 0 to 10, how much fatigue, tiredness, or exhaustion do you experience?

None		Mild		Moderate		Severe		Very Severe	
0	1	2	3	4	5	6	7	8	9	10

How much of a problem is sore throat?

None		Mild		Moderate		Severe		Very Severe	
0	1	2	3	4	5	6	7	8	9	10

How severe are headaches?

None		Mild		Moderate		Severe		Very Severe	
0	1	2	3	4	5	6	7	8	9	10

How much of a problem is aching of the eyes, blurry vision, or light sensitivity?

None		Mild		Moderate		Severe		Very Severe
0	1	2	3	4	5	6	7	8	9	10

How much of a problem is abdominal pain, bloating, or gas?

None		Mild		Moderate		Severe		Very Severe
0	1	2	3	4	5	6	7	8	9	10

How much of a problem is pain in your lymph nodes?

None		Mild		Moderate		Severe		Very Severe
0	1	2	3	4	5	6	7	8	9	10

How much of a problem is depression, mood changes, or panic attacks?

None		Mild		Moderate		Severe		Very Severe
0	1	2	3	4	5	6	7	8	9	10

How much of a problem is pain or aching in your muscles?

None		Mild		Moderate		Severe		Very Severe
0	1	2	3	4	5	6	7	8	9	10

How much of a problem is memory loss or difficulty concentrating?

None		Mild		Moderate		Severe		Very Severe
0	1	2	3	4	5	6	7	8	9	10

How much of a problem is poor sleep, insomnia, or waking unrefreshed?

None		Mild		Moderate		Severe		Very Severe
0	1	2	3	4	5	6	7	8	9	10

How much concern is numbness, tingling, dizziness, or balance problems?

None		Mild		Moderate		Severe		Very Severe
0	1	2	3	4	5	6	7	8	9	10

How much of a problem is pain in your joints?

None		Mild		Moderate		Severe		Very Severe
0	1	2	3	4	5	6	7	8	9	10

A graph is constructed with lines extending from the center like spokes on a wheel. The severity of each symptom is marked on the spokes. The 0 is at the center of the wheel, and 10 is at the circumference. The order of symptoms on the spokes is important, as seen below.

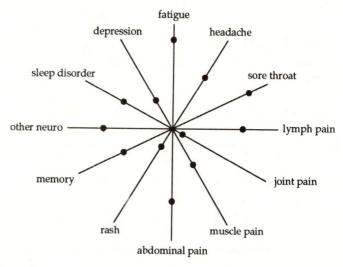

Figure 9–1

Let us assume that a hypothetical patient with moderate CFIDS has all twelve symptoms and marks their severity as follows: fatigue = 8; headache = 5; sore throat = 7; lymph node pain = 6; joint pain = 1; muscle pain = 3; abdominal pain = 6; rash = 2; memory and concentration loss = 5; numbness, tingling, and weakness (other neuro) = 6; sleep disorder = 5; depression = 3. These points marked on the graph are shown in the preceding illustration.

The symptom severity on each of the twelve spokes is now connected, creating a pattern of symptoms that can be assessed visually. However, of greater importance is that the area under this pattern can be calculated, giving us an objective number that reflects both the pattern and severity of symptoms. The total area is the sum of each of the twelve separate triangles. For example, the area of the "fatigue-headache" triangle is calculated by multiplying fatigue times headache and dividing the product by four: (8)(5)/4 = 10. The total area is then calculated by adding the area of each triangle. A radial plot with the symptom severity marked would look like this:

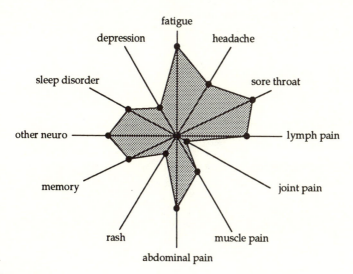

Figure 9-2

In this particular example the shaded area has an area of 67.25, which is in the average range for patients with CFIDS. The total area is a function not only of the number but of the pattern of symptoms adjacent to each other. For example, if a particular symptom is missing—that is, has a severity of 0—then the area of both adjoining triangles is zero. Let us calculate the radial plot for a patient with six severe symptoms, each with a severity of 10, but none of the six symptoms is next to another symptom: fatigue = 10; headache = 0; sore throat = 10; lymph node pain = 0; joint pain = 10; muscle pain = 0; abdominal pain = 10;

rash = 0; attention and memory loss = 10; paresthesias (other neuro) = 0; sleep disorder = 10; depression = 0. In this patient, the total area of the radial plot is zero.

Because the total area is dependent on both the severity and the pattern of symptoms, one possibility of this system is to differentiate CFIDS from other illnesses, such as depression. A patient with primary depression might have the following symptoms: fatigue = 7; depression = 9; sleep disorder = 4; headache = 5; abdominal pain = 7; memory and concentration loss = 5. In this patient the pattern would appear visually different from CFIDS, and the radial plot score, 35.75, would be much less than in typical CFIDS.

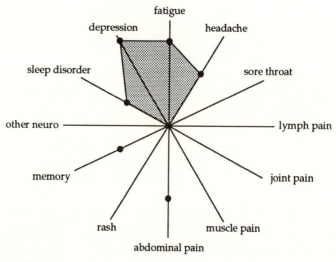

Figure 9–3

Conclusions

Establishing disability has been a nightmare for patients with CFIDS, primarily because of the medical debate as to whether this illness is real. As the debate continued, patients lost their jobs, their insurance, and their savings, and yet were unable to receive disability benefits. The situation may be changing. Recognition of the illness by the Centers for Disease Control and the Social Security Administration has allowed some patients to win their disability claim.

But the process is difficult, and many patients do not have the strength for a prolonged, isolated legal struggle. CFIDS patients who are disabled should receive benefits as with any other medical condition, and they should be aided by the physician. It may be frustrating and difficult for a physician to treat people with CFIDS, but it is inexcusable to abandon patients when they seek disability compensation. All too often abandoned already by friends, employers, and sometimes family, patients with CFIDS who are abandoned by their physician will certainly be abandoned by their country.

PART 4

Treatment of CFIDS

CHAPTER 10

Prognosis or Outcome

It is impossible to begin a discussion of treatment of an illness without first knowing something about its natural course or history. If an illness were one that spontaneously resolved after a short time, we would judge a treatment on the basis of whether it shortened the time to resolution. If an illness invariably progressed, however, a treatment would be considered successful if it merely slowed the progression.

A number of patients have told me that they started to feel better when they began a certain treatment. This information can be interpreted in a few different ways: (1) Were the patients spontaneously about to improve, which was coincident with the time of beginning a certain medicine? (2) Did the treatment affect them positively but not help other patients with the same illness (idiosyncratic response)? (3) Was it the treatment that effected the positive change, or was it something else such as lifestyle modification? Before assessing the possibilities of treatment, let us look at the usual course of CFIDS—its "natural history"—to observe what is likely without treatment.

Cure Versus Improvement

There is considerable debate concerning the prognosis of patients with CFIDS, and unfortunately at the present time we do not have enough data to answer the questions accurately. However, we can make several general statements. The majority of patients with CFIDS are doing well five years after becoming ill. Some of the improvement may be due to lessening the severity of symptoms, some is due to loss of fear about the disease, and some is due to accommodation or adjustment in lifestyle. Regardless of the reason, the overall prognosis is good for the majority of patients (Marshall 91; Shafran 91; Bell 93, unpublished observations).

If, however, we take complete cure as the goal, relatively few patients actually achieve it. Of those patients who are doing well five years after having had CFIDS, many relate residual decreases in exercise tolerance, and mild symptoms that appear to be related to their previous CFIDS. The symptoms are exacerbated during periods of stress and minor illnesses.

Therefore, we must be careful in defining the clinical outcome, something that has not been well done in the earlier outbreaks of CFIDS. Complete resolution of all symptoms would imply that the illness is cured and that the basic pathologic processes are now absent. It is quite different from "doing well with minor symptoms," which implies that although a patient is functioning well, the pathologic process is continuing.

When a patient's symptoms persist for five years, it is unlikely the illness is going to improve much after that. If there is going to be resolution, it seems to happen within five years. As a corollary, if a patient does have resolution of symptoms and returns to normal exercise tolerance, it is rare for the illness to return.

*H*istorical Prognosis

Perhaps the greatest disappointment in reviewing the reports of earlier outbreaks is the paucity of data on rate and degree of recovery. It would be of tremendous value to see what has happened to all the patients of a certain outbreak twenty years ago and know how many recovered completely; how many still have mild, moderate, or severe symptoms; and how many developed other diseases, such as cancer or multiple sclerosis. Unfortunately, we may have to wait for another twenty years to get these answers, but at least the literature does give us some hints.

One common thread that runs through the literature is the lack of case fatalities and the symptomatic improvement over time.

Bearing in mind that different standards are used by different investigators, the overall impression is that the majority of patients, up to 80 percent, are functioning well after two years of illness. Other illnesses may have complicated the course of CFIDS, but these are not commented on in any of the studies.

Six months after the acute onset in an epidemic in Punta Gorda, Florida, five of twelve patients were still confined to bed at least one day a week. At eighteen months all were functioning well. In the Los Angeles County Hospital epidemic, 24 percent missed at least five months of work, followed by improvement. In London's Royal Free epidemic, follow-up statistics varied as widely as the original diagnoses. Some said that 43 percent of patients received inpatient care for more than a month, and that after two years all but four patients had a complete recovery except for residual symptoms of depression (Behan 88a). Others state that a large majority have persisting fatigue and other symptoms, and that a small number continue to have, twenty years later, "relapsing multifocal CNS disease" (Thomas 87).

An epidemic in Alaska was followed carefully, and all 175 patients were re-evaluated after two years (Goldenberg 88). Symptoms were present in 110, or 63 percent of these patients. The Iceland epidemic was reviewed six years later, and although all patients had returned to work, only 13 percent considered themselves completely free of symptoms.

One of the great difficulties in the previous medical studies on CFIDS has been the inability to compare groups of patients from one study to another. Just as different investigators have used different standards for diagnosing the illness, different standards are used in monitoring the outcome. One of the most important tasks in the next few years is the development of standardized instruments for diagnosis and clinical staging. Without this standardization we will continue to be bewildered by the long-term outcome.

Fatal Complications

Are there fatal complications of CFIDS? This question has also generated debate among researchers. Although I have not studied the question in detail, my feeling is that the primary fatal complication is suicide. Patients are often very ill, but their symptoms are trivialized. Implications or direct accusations of malingering are common. Patients become isolated not only from the medical community but from their family and friends because they are accused of imagining symptoms. The despair grows if physicians are unwilling to discuss symptoms, dismissing everything the patient says as a manifestation of depression. The poor recognition of this symptom complex by the medical community is the greatest risk factor for fatal complications in patients with this illness.

In addition to the depression caused from these external events, there are very real problems with mood changes, paranoia, and organic depression. Patients commonly discuss periods in their life when they were close to suicide, and after struggling with depression some do kill themselves. At this point in the research on CFIDS there are no statistics available to study this issue.

Another potentially fatal complication of CFIDS is the light-headedness or syncope that occurs, frequently at the onset of the illness. This is usually of minor significance, except when patients have fainting spells without warning while driving, which obviously can be fatal regardless of the cause. Fortunately, however, although CFIDS patients may have dizzy spells, actual loss of consciousness is quite rare.

But let me emphasize that in and of itself, CFIDS is not fatal.

Factors Influencing Recovery

Several specific factors are related to the speed and degree of recovery: (1) type or pattern of onset, acute versus gradual; (2) age at the time of onset; (3) pattern of relapses; and (4) prominence of neurologic symptoms. The following discussion on the prognosis of CFIDS is drawn from observations only, and no comprehensive studies have been published. It is possible that several years from now we will have an entirely different view of the prognosis of this illness.

Pattern of Onset

The most common CFIDS patient is the thirty- to forty-year-old adult who was entirely well before an acute onset of an influenza-like or mononucleosis-like illness. In the majority of patients who fit the diagnostic criteria presently available, the clinical course is marked by gradual improvement beginning within one year of onset and continuing until the symptoms are either resolved or much improved three or four years later. The course is rarely smooth; there may be marked relapses and remissions during this time period. The clinical course described in Figure 10–1 shows acute onset with severe symptoms and gradual improvement over time. Although patients in this category may be quite ill initially, they have a good chance of recovery.

In epidemic areas, CFIDS is recognized more readily, and patients with milder cases are diagnosed. In these areas the overall outcome is better than in nonepidemic areas, where only the most severe cases are recognized. For example, in the Lyndonville, New York, epidemic, 104 patients met the severity criteria of 50 percent activity reduction for at least six months. But at least another hundred people had the same pattern of symptoms, although milder. This latter group, the majority of whom had acute onset, recovered

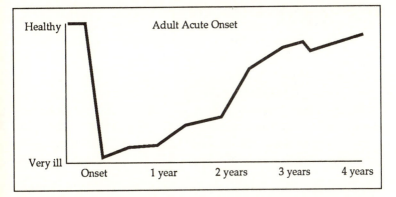

Figure 10–1: The most common course of CFIDS in adults, with an acute flulike onset followed by slow and steady recovery over the next several years.

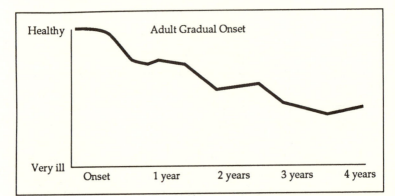

Figure 10–2: Gradual onset of CFIDS with prolonged course over years. Patients with this type of onset seem to be less ill than those with acute onset, but also seem to have less chance of complete recovery. This pattern is more common in younger children.

quite well. If we assume that CFIDS can occur with different degrees of severity, we can generalize and say that the milder the course, the better the overall chance of recovery.

Whether the symptoms will recur in the future after an apparent recovery is not known. I know of three adults who were ill as teenagers, recovered completely, and subsequently developed CFIDS for a second time up to twenty years later. In general, however, the recurrence of CFIDS after recovery of full exercise tolerance for one year is extremely rare.

The second onset pattern is shown in Figure 10–2 and is the gradual or insidious onset, with symptoms appearing gradually over months or years. These patients are rarely as ill as those with acute onset and do not have the full range of symptoms initially. However, although not as ill, they also seem to have less chance of recovery within the same time frame. Those with a gradual onset of symptoms are more likely to experience the symptoms for many years, perhaps indefinitely.

Age at Onset

The pattern of gradual onset of symptoms is of great concern in children who develop CFIDS before the age of ten. Children frequently have gradual onset and do not appear to resolve their symptoms as rapidly as adults with acute onset. Moreover, of the many patients I have seen who have had symptoms of CFIDS for fifteen or twenty years, the majority of them first became ill during childhood. However, the symptoms are generally not as severe as those in patients with an acute onset.

For teenagers with an acute onset of symptoms, the outlook is good, and perhaps the majority will recover to normal activity. The more severe the onset, however, the less chance of recovery. In the adolescents I have studied with CFIDS, over half with an acute onset have recovered and were either completely well or nearly well three years after the onset of their symptoms.

Overall the prognosis for children with CFIDS is good. In part this may be because they adapt to a certain level of functioning more readily than do adults. They may not actually resolve their symptoms more readily than adults, but children function better because they are more flexible and adaptable.

However, data are lacking in all the present research. Diagnostic confusion, syndrome definitions, lack of funding, and a general lack of interest on the part of physicians have contributed to the present lack of information. Despite CFIDS being so common, we know remarkably little about its outcome.

Pattern of Relapses

A third factor that seems to influence the chance of recovery is the pattern of relapses within the first year or two of the illness. An ominous course for a patient with CFIDS, fortunately less common, is a pattern characterized by no relapses and remissions. If a patient has good days and good weeks, followed by severe relapses lasting for a few weeks, the overall chance of recovery is good. If there are any periods of return to near normal activity, even though followed by marked ups and downs, I am encouraged. The pattern of every day being the same, with the same symptoms and exactly the same degree of activity limitation, is more worrisome.

It is just the opposite of what patients would expect. Patients are upset that they had been feeling pretty well and then had a

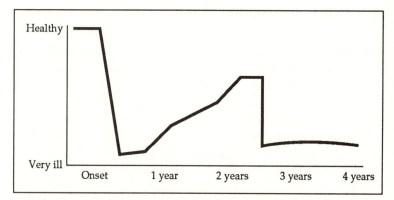

Figure 10–3: A rare pattern consisting of change from the optimistic recovery after acute onset to the steady, severe course, devoid of fluctuations associated with a poor long-term prognosis.

severe relapse. But I believe that this pattern is more encouraging than a course characterized by a monotonous sameness of symptoms and limitation day after day.

Occasionally a patient has a typical acute onset and begins a slow, steady, modest recovery a year or so after onset, a pattern like Figure 10–1 that is quite encouraging. However, for no apparent reason, the pattern changes with a severe and extended relapse, followed by a course with no fluctuations, relapses, or remissions (Figure 10–3). This patient would seem to have switched from an optimistic course to the more ominous, and the reasons are not clear. Fortunately, this does not happen often. The rare patient who fits this picture should have a complete reevaluation of the illness with an attempt to determine the cause of the relapse. In particular, I would look carefully for the development of a separate illness that has caused the change in course. It is because this pattern is so rare that suspicion is aroused.

Prominence of Neurologic Symptoms

Another factor that seems to influence the overall outcome is the prominence of neurologic symptoms. Virtually all patients have neurologic symptoms, but for some they are clearly more severe.

Patients who have persistent, very severe neurologic symptoms are more likely to have persistence of their illness.

During the evaluation of symptoms in CFIDS, it is helpful to determine the order of what symptoms cause the patient the greatest problem. For example, one patient is most distressed by fatigue. Another has frequent sore throat and lymph gland swelling, which, along with the tiredness, is the most severe. Both of these patients, on questioning, also describe confusion, difficulty paying attention, and memory problems. But their likelihood of recovery seems to be greater than the patient who says that the neurologic symptoms are more disabling than the fatigue or sore throats.

The most ominous pattern is a combination of severe neurologic symptoms in a patient who, two years after onset, has no day-to-day fluctuations. Every day is marked by the same headaches, dizziness, confusion, memory loss, and exhaustion: there are no "good days" and "bad days." This course is marked by its severity, lack of fluctuations, and lack of improvement over the three- or four-year time frame. Fortunately, it is less common.

Conclusion

The research needs are enormous and obvious. We should be looking for biologic markers to distinguish patients who are more and less likely to recover. What is the role of genetic factors? What role do emotional complications play in the recovery or lack of recovery? What is the role of treatment in recovery?

What we do not know far outweighs what we do know about the prognosis of CFIDS. But, having been involved in an epidemic, I have been encouraged by the large number of victims who have either fully recovered or recovered to a nearly normal functional state and are leading productive lives. I have also been encouraged by how few people have developed other serious diseases or complications. I am even more hopeful that with newer treatment regimens, the outlook will change completely over the coming years.

This certainly does not imply that CFIDS is a benign disease. Even people who recover completely may have had a three-year period of agony in their lives—a lapse in their health that led them, their family, and their physicians to doubt their honesty and sanity; a period of amnesia during which life was put on hold, families separated, dreams shattered, security lost; a nightmare that has redirected the course of their lives. The lucky ones can rebuild, start fresh. Those not so lucky, like returning war veterans, will never recover completely, even if physical health is restored.

CHAPTER 11

General Treatment Principles

*A*t the present time there is no cure for CFIDS. No single medication or treatment can consistently make the symptoms disappear and activity return to normal. This does not mean that people with CFIDS do not get better, just that we do not know how to make this improvement happen with treatment. On the other hand, I have heard physicians say that CFIDS cannot be treated. Although there may not be a cure for CFIDS now, it is incorrect to say that nothing can be done. There are many illnesses for which a cure is not at hand, yet treatments are available to improve symptoms.

It is important to remember the natural history of CFIDS presented in the preceding chapter. Many, perhaps most, people who develop the illness improve or recover with time. This recovery will either occur or not occur depending on the severity of the illness, and I do not believe that it is related to the specific treatment employed. It is important to maintain this perspective, and treatment strategies should be dominated by common sense, enhancing coping ability, and a view toward the future.

*T*reatment of Symptoms or Treatment of Underlying Cause?

One basic issue to be understood is the difference between treating symptoms of an illness and treating its cause. With respect to treatment, CFIDS can be compared to rheumatoid arthritis. Numerous treatments are available that help patients in the management of pain and joint stiffness, but the underlying cause of the disease cannot be cured. We may not know how to remove or cure the underlying cause of CFIDS, but there are many treatments that may help individual symptoms. Fortunately, the symptomatic treatments available for CFIDS are usually known and available to practicing physicians.

One of the problems the physician faces is knowing how to approach treatment in general, and it is in this area that the patient must help. A patient will have many symptoms, all of which cause distress and discomfort, and for some of these, treatments are available. But it is not wise to treat a patient with CFIDS with ten different medications, since there are certain to be side effects and drug interactions. The patient must decide which symptoms cause the greatest disability, pain, and/or limitation, and help direct treatment toward that particular symptom. Again, a commonsense approach is important.

Patients with mild to moderate symptoms and activity limitation frequently have a strong placebo response. This statement may horrify and insult patients because it is often interpreted to mean that no illness is present. CFIDS is certainly a real disease, and as with other serious illnesses a placebo response exists and must be taken into account. However, I have noticed relatively little placebo response in patients very ill with CFIDS.

I can remember a time when I became very excited about a medication I believed would improve the symptom of fatigue. I prescribed this medication to my patients and my enthusiasm was obvious. Patients seemed to do well on the medication, and I was further encouraged. However, I soon noticed that the overall degree of disability did not appear to change. That is, although patients stated that they felt better, they were not able to improve their level of activity. I performed a medication trial in which patients were unable to tell which was the exciting new drug and which was an inert substance, or placebo. To my dismay, there was no difference in symptom response between the two. This meant that it was not really the medication that was making patients feel better, it was their hope and my enthusiasm. The medication I was using "worked" for two reasons: the patients' hopes had soared because they were being treated, and my enthusiasm gave them support and improved their ability to cope.

Treatment of Trigger Agent

Let us return for a moment to the concept of the trigger agent. In CFIDS, treatment of a trigger agent would not be the same as treatment of the underlying cause of the illness. If the illness is expressed because of the trigger agent, then treatment of this agent may improve symptoms. Yet because the underlying cause is still present, some symptoms persist and the illness is not cured. Another trigger agent may come along and exacerbate the symptoms again. However, if the concept of trigger agent is correct, then it makes sense to improve symptoms as much as possible by eliminating the factors that cause exacerbation.

The trigger agent concept in CFIDS is no different from that in many other diseases, especially those involving immune system abnormalities. If a patient is feeling poorly because of an underlying disease (cancer, for example) and develops a strep throat, this secondary infection will markedly worsen the symptoms, more so than a strep throat in a healthy person. Effective treatment for the strep throat will improve the symptoms while not affecting the underlying malignancy. In CFIDS there may be certain infections that either trigger the illness or worsen the symptoms, and many of these infections are treatable.

Patients state that certain medications, such as gamma globulin or Acyclovir (to be discussed later), may improve symptoms, yet large medication trials have not consistently shown them to be effective treatments. While the placebo response is a possibility, it is also possible that in these patients the medication is directed against the trigger agent and not the underlying cause of CFIDS.

With these factors in mind, let us turn to the many questions that treatment of CFIDS poses: What are the general measures that will improve function and lessen symptom severity? What is the role of nonmedication treatments? How much, if any, exercise is appropriate? What types of symptoms should be treated first? Because CFIDS patients are sensitive to medications, should they "tough out" the early days of a treatment, despite discomfort? How do medications interact in CFIDS? How can we be sure that treatments being used will ultimately not worsen the illness?

*T*ypes of Treatment

Patients frequently forget about nonmedication measures, and this is a mistake. I believe that the most important treatments available at the present time are not related to drugs. The basis of CFIDS treatment is the following: learn, be realistic, and cope as well as you can. Many inexpensive, safe, and possibly helpful treatment measures can be tried independently by the patient without a physician's guidance, measures usually taken for granted. Guided by common sense, the patient can try these measures, observe the effects on themselves, and evaluate their usefulness.

I am fully in support of nontraditional remedies for symptom treatment as long as they stay within the bounds of common sense. Acupuncture, yoga, meditation, visualization, herbal remedies, and many other treatments, although I do not understand them, may improve symptoms in individual cases without serious risk and should be explored. However, when expectations are too high or the expense too great, or when hope has murdered common sense, disaster may result. As with pharmacologic treatment, learn, be realistic, and cope as well as you can.

My treatment preferences are as follows, presented in order of importance.

Education About the Nature of CFIDS

I feel that the single greatest treatment offered by the physician is an accurate diagnosis. Patients may travel from physician to physician and receive a variety of diagnoses ranging from possible multiple sclerosis to possible depression, yet they know that none of these diagnoses is correct. They know depression could not cause the lymph node pain, and they could not have lupus if their lupus tests are always negative. Perhaps the greatest insult to the patient is that on initial evaluation, the concern around dangerous possibilities is so great that the physician orders numerous tests, including biopsies. Yet when these tests are negative, the same physician says that the symptoms are probably due to minor depression or even that there is nothing wrong at all. Patients are acutely aware of these inconsistencies, and are left with the fear that something is terribly wrong, even fatal, but that the physician cannot find it. Therefore, patients seek multiple opinions and receive a bewildering array of diagnoses.

When the diagnosis of CFIDS is made after a careful history of symptoms, complete physical examination, and elimination of other possible diagnoses, the patient feels a sense of relief. Education concerning the nature of CFIDS brings empowerment and the decreased anxiety stemming from no longer facing the unknown. Their illness is not fatal and is likely to improve with time.

Only with an accurate diagnosis can patients begin to learn about their illness, and in this regard CFIDS is again no different from other illnesses. Anxiety begins to fade, and the process of accommodation begins. If the patient is lucky, the symptoms will improve with time, perhaps disappear completely. If the patient is not lucky, the symptoms will persist, but the process of acceptance has begun. Life can go on despite the illness. Without an accurate diagnosis, everything becomes more difficult, and it is possible that because of added stress and fear of the unknown, the symptoms and disability become worse.

Appropriate Activity Limitation and Lifestyle Adjustments

After diagnosis the first treatment strategy revolves around appropriate rest and lifestyle adjustment. CFIDS is characterized by, indeed almost defined by, the worsening of symptoms with exertion, exercise or activity, and sometimes even mental activity. Therefore patients quickly learn out of necessity to rest frequently during the day. This rest may take the form of lying on a couch or actually sleeping, and the day's plans usually revolve around the rest periods.

Every patient is different in this regard. They experiment and learn what they can tolerate and what makes the flulike symptoms worse. What may be an effective rest program for one patient may be inappropriate for another. People with CFIDS should try different patterns and observe how they feel. Furthermore, because the illness has relapses and remissions, the amount of rest needed during the day vary. Patients should recognize this and be flexible.

On a given day, an average patient has a few hours during which he or she feels relatively well, and although the symptoms never entirely disappear, they may abate enough so that some activity, such as shopping, school, or even work, is possible. With experience, the patient may plan activities around this period, called the "activity window," usually in the early afternoon.

Acceptance of the Limitations Imposed by the Illness

Only through acceptance of the physical limitations imposed by CFIDS can a patient function effectively within them. Denial of the limitations will cause chaos, as overexertion will precipitate relapses, followed by bed rest, followed by more chaos. The acceptance of limitations is related to education concerning CFIDS, a process that all patients can achieve by listening to their bodies. With acceptance of the limitations, overall function usually improves.

Some patients feel that acceptance of the limitations is the same as giving up. It is not. Accepting today's limitations does not imply that tomorrow's will be the same. In fact, many patients with "moderate severity" CFIDS have even day-to-day variation of the activity limitation. By monitoring the degree of limitation carefully, the patient can maximize overall activity and reduce frustration.

I think it is as much of a mistake to overrest as it is to overdo. Although rest lessens symptom severity somewhat, I do not believe it will cure the illness, and there comes a point where excessive rest is self-defeating. It creates false hope as the CFIDS patient sacrifices the limited activity available on the altar of expected cure.

Finding a middle ground that satisfies many individual factors is best. Each patient must find his or her own unique and individual middle ground; a physician can only support the process.

Stress Reduction

Stress does not cause CFIDS but, as with any illness, can exacerbate symptoms. It is common sense that when you feel ill, the last thing you need is stress. Unfortunately, this is often just what the doctor ordered. By not understanding CFIDS and implying that the patient can "snap out of it," the physician creates an additional burden of stress. The patient then attempts to ignore the illness, usually overdoes, and then the symptoms become worse. The problem here is that then the patient will overcompensate and restrict activity too much. This also causes additional stress because of family or financial concerns.

Also, stress is unpleasant. It is unpleasant for everyone, but particularly for someone who is feeling ill. Nearly all techniques designed for stress reduction may be appropriate for someone with CFIDS. Meditation, visualization, and relaxation techniques are wonderful, yet take some effort on the part of the patient to accomplish.

Sleep Hygiene

Disturbed sleep in one form or another is a universal symptom of CFIDS. Some patients have hypersomnolence, some have insomnia or easy waking during the night. But nearly all describe waking unrefreshed in the morning. The anticipated restorative effect of sleep has been stripped away. Some researchers have felt that the sleep disorder may be the most important aspect of CFIDS, and that many of the other symptoms arise from functional sleep deprivation, even though fifteen hours were spent supposedly asleep.

Sleep hygiene techniques are methods to improve the quality of sleep. They may be as simple as adjusting the temperature and noise level of your sleeping area to more complex methods of positioning during sleep to improve air exchange. Perhaps your mattress needs replacing. Perhaps you need better shades to keep out the light from the street lamp outside. There are many approaches to sleep hygiene, and several popular books have been written to educate on this subject. It is a factor that needs to be considered by the patient with CFIDS.

Exercise Within the Bounds of Common Sense

In the past, physicians have assumed that the fatigue of CFIDS is related to depression, and one characteristic of the fatigue of depression is that it improves with exercise. Thus, physicians have been recommending that their patients take a brisk walk around the block every day or maybe take up jogging. Patients with primary depression may do well with this regimen, but patients with CFIDS stare at their physician with a look of disbelief. Many try it, only to find that it worsens the symptoms. To the patient, the symptom worsening confirms two things: (1) that the physician has absolutely no idea of what he or she is talking about, and (2) that the illness is not primary depression.

Yet there is a role for exercise in the treatment of this illness. Patients describe a point at which they can perform an activity and still feel relatively well. If they push beyond this point they begin to develop the flulike discomfort or malaise. I think every patient should learn to recognize this point and try to exercise up to, but not beyond, it. Again, this point is different for every patient and may fluctuate within the same patient, depending on relapses and remissions. Common sense is the key. If a patient is beginning to feel waves of exhaustion after doing the dishes, it is time to rest. On another day it might be possible to walk around the block. For some, more vigorous exercise is possible, keeping in mind that point at which the achiness, lymph node pain, and exhaustion will start.

Can exercise harm a patient with CFIDS? Of the professional athletes with CFIDS I have seen, several were improving nicely and decided to get into shape again. Because of their well-developed self-discipline, they were able to push themselves despite feeling poorly. In several instances severe relapses ensued, causing marked regression. I have never seen an athlete try this twice.

Does exertion worsen the illness as well as the symptoms? At this point there have been no good medical studies to document the answer to this question, but I believe that, within the limits of common sense, it does not. For example, a man with moderate symptoms may be invited to a friend's wedding. The patient knows that if he goes it will make him feel quite sick for a week or two. Yet it is an important event. Should he go? He must weigh the advantages of going against the expected worsening of symptoms, and every patient approaches such a decision differently. I do not think that exertion will worsen the illness or prolong recovery, if it is going to occur. The patient may feel quite ill for a week or two after the wedding, but he has accomplished something important. The satisfaction of having participated in the friend's wedding may be worth the temporary worsening of symptoms.

However, common sense and a good sense of balance are important. People with CFIDS need to become accurate observers of themselves and their abilities, and then objectively decide on what course of action to take. Although it is not good to push beyond certain limits, it is also not good to be paralyzed by the fear of temporarily worsening the symptoms.

Nutritional Supplementation Within the Bounds of Common Sense

There has been a great deal of controversy and confusion over the role of nutrition in the treatment of CFIDS, a subject that I will touch on only briefly because I lack knowledge of it. Many patients state that they feel better when they eat a nutritious diet, avoiding sugars and junk food. I have heard this consistently and have little doubt that it is true. Patients have also told me that they became completely well after starting certain diets. Unfortunately, this happens only rarely, and there appears to be great variety among diets that have been helpful. My interpretation is that these patients were in the process of improving and happened to start a certain diet at the same time. When I have tried these same diets in other patients I have not noticed a consistent response. I have no doubt that good nutrition and even modest vitamin supplements make sense whenever a person is ill, whether with CFIDS or any other disease. To date, however, I have not been convinced that any specific diet can cure the illness.

Many patients have food sensitivities, and will notice that when they eat certain food groups their symptoms worsen. I think that this represents not true food allergies, but rather a difficulty in processing and handling certain foods. Perhaps the most common offending food group is dairy products. In general, I recommend that my patients observe for worsening of symptoms with foods, and if this worsening is consistent, then avoid the foods responsible.

Again, the treatment is common sense. Eat nutritious foods in all food groups, take reasonable vitamin and mineral supplementation, and avoid foods that make you feel worse. Be careful of weight gain. A patient with CFIDS does not burn off many calories and must watch food intake.

Support and Understanding from Physicians, Family, and Friends

Support should be available to people who require it, regardless of cause. With CFIDS, this support is particularly important. The limitations of CFIDS are so complex and life is disrupted so completely that help with activities, shopping, and managing daily life is usually necessary. The amount of support required depends on the severity of the illness.

More important than the help with daily chores is understanding. The confusion experienced by the CFIDS patient is enormous. Suddenly an active, productive person becomes a helpless invalid, diagnosed with a strange illness, yet because the person looks well, no one believes that he or she is ill. The patient struggles to come to terms with the life disruption and the constant feeling of being sick. Support from family and friends is crucial. The patient with CFIDS needs the time and space to come to accept this new definition of daily life.

However, the patient with CFIDS should not abuse or manipulate the support offered. No one likes to hear complaining or whining; it makes the listener feel inadequate, hopeless, even angry. The CFIDS patient needs to be considerate of friends and family and, while not being dishonest, should hold the incessant details of discomfort private.

Psychotherapy is often helpful for patients with CFIDS. I do not think that it is curative, but patients with CFIDS usually need to sort out hundreds of conflicting feelings and emotions.

Physiotherapy is another form of physical support that may be of value. Patients may have a temporary improvement of joint and muscle symptoms with physiotherapy techniques, a phenomenon well studied in fibromyalgia. Again common sense is important, and if heat, passive stretching exercises, and other physiotherapy techniques improve the symptoms and reduce stress, I would continue with them. Physiotherapy is safe and should be considered a symptomatic treatment, since it is unlikely to affect the underlying disease process.

Pharmacologic Symptomatic Treatment

It is this final area in our discussion that many patients wish to jump to first, and the next chapter will discuss the specifics. But I would emphasize its place in the management of CFIDS; it cannot magically solve all the problems of the illness. Furthermore, the best results with pharmacologic treatments have occurred when the preceding suggestions have been considered and digested. Relatively little is gained with medications when they are not accompanied by other methods of treatment.

CHAPTER 12

An Approach to Medication

*I*t is unrealistic to expect a medication or two to solve the difficulties imposed by CFIDS, but they can be useful as a part of the overall treatment plan, and can be specifically targeted against certain symptoms. Here it is important for the physician and patient to work together as a team. The patient must examine which symptoms should be treated and the physician must dig into the armamentarium of medications. With a cautious, realistic approach and a little luck, life will be better for the patient.

There are two general approaches to the use of medications in the treatment of CFIDS. One is to attempt to improve overall function and general activity, to create stamina and a sense of increased energy. The other is to reduce the severity of certain symptoms such as headache, joint pain, and difficulty thinking. They are independent problems, and ultimately any treatment that accomplishes the first will probably prove to be acting on the underlying cause of the illness. Unfortunately, it is the more difficult of the two approaches. For the purposes of this discussion, improving overall function will be discussed under the symptom of fatigue, but they are not really the same.

General Principles with Medications

A number of general principles specific to CFIDS are useful to mention before delving into the drugs themselves. Many patients have had bad experiences with medications and are reluctant to attempt them further. However, with these principles in mind, some of these bad experiences can be avoided.

1. *Monitor responses carefully.* I use a method of rating both symptoms and activity on a daily basis in order to assess the effectiveness of symptomatic treatment. The nature and severity of symptoms are complex and memories fade quickly, so unless there is a dramatic response, it will blend into the haze of the past and become useless in directing future symptomatic treatment. A copy of the symptom rating form that I use is included in appendix 1 and may be freely reproduced and used by doctors and patients alike.

2. *If a symptomatic medicine is not helping, don't use it.* At present I view all the medications I try, with the single exception of a vitamin supplement, as symptomatic treatment. I wish these pharmacologic aids were changing the underlying nature of the illness, but I do not see this occurring. If a symptomatic treatment does not help the symptoms within the time frame characteristic for it, don't use it. And any benefit of a medication should be obvious. If there is doubt about effectiveness, then it probably is not working. The medication can always be stopped and restarted to assess whether it was helping a particular symptom or group of symptoms. A severely disabled patient with CFIDS is usually on many medications; my first step in treatment is to stop most of them.

3. *The symptoms will fluctuate in intensity even without treatment.* If you start a symptomatic treatment, you need not stay on it for the next twenty years. Some symptoms, such as pressure headaches, come and go. If there is symptomatic improvement, try removing the medication. Be sure that the medicine you are taking is doing something. There is no point in taking a medication if the symptom happened to go away by coincidence.

4. *Use medications least likely to do harm or cause unpleasant reactions.* If we were removing the underlying cause of CFIDS, it would be worthwhile to take risks. But we are only treating symptoms,

and it is prudent to use safe and well-known medications. If a patient is desperate, then some risks can be taken but only with a complete and full explanation of the risks involved. Fortunately, nearly all the medications used in the treatment of CFIDS are safe. The hoped-for benefit must be weighed against the risks of a particular treatment. Use common sense. For example, the benefits of taking a bath outweigh the risk of slipping in the bathtub.

5. *Use caution and low doses.* Many patients with CFIDS are sensitive to medications. Bad responses often can be avoided by starting at very low doses and gradually increasing. The tricyclic antidepressants are an example of this; many people will say they are allergic to a certain medication because of a bad reaction to the standard dose. However, a smaller dose may still be quite effective in symptomatic treatment. Do not confuse drug allergy with a bad response. A true drug allergy means that you should not attempt to try that class of medications in the future.

6. *Introduce or change only one medicine at a time.* Because we are looking at symptom responses, it is essential to observe the symptoms closely. If you make more than one change in medications, you will not know the reason for any change in symptoms. Be sure that you will be able to identify the cause of changes.

*T*he Groups of Medications

Medications are grouped on the basis of their chemical properties and the symptoms they attempt to treat. Usually the effect seen with one medication in a group is shared by all medicines in that group. For example, a person who is allergic to penicillin would also be allergic to ampicillin, amoxicillin, and all other drugs of the class.

In CFIDS there is some variation of effect with different drugs within a class, and cautious attempts to try other medications within a class are appropriate assuming there is no allergy. In the following discussion drugs will be cited by their chemical (generic) names and brand names will appear in brackets [ ]. There is usually no value in switching brand names since they are the same drug. Sometimes, however, one brand may be more convenient than another.

Sometimes, several symptom groups may respond to a specific category of medications. If a patient has several disturbing symptoms within a symptom group, then a single medication might have multiple uses. Try to maximize the benefits with the fewest number of medications.

Analgesics

Plain old aspirin is my first choice as a treatment agent for CFIDS. Patients may be dismayed at this because virtually all have tried it, long before they even went to the doctor's office, and have been discouraged. But if taken carefully it may help. It is most effective in patients with prominent joint and muscle pain, headache, lymph node pain, and general aching and is less effective in patients with prominent fatigue, nausea, and neurologic symptoms.

One trick worth trying is borrowed from the long experience with aspirin in treating rheumatoid arthritis. Instead of waiting for the symptoms to become severe, try taking it on a regular basis, spacing it out during the day to maintain effective blood levels. If joint pain and stiffness are particularly bad in the morning, try taking aspirin at bedtime.

Like every medication, aspirin has drawbacks. Bleeding from the gastrointestinal tract can be caused by aspirin, so monitoring with routine checks for anemia is necessary. Black stools or any blood in the stool would imply a significant amount of bleeding. Stomach and duodenal ulcers can be caused by aspirin, as well as heartburn and worsening of abdominal pain. Buffered aspirin may help these problems somewhat, but does not eliminate them. And because aspirin acts as a blood thinner, it should not be taken with anticoagulants. If you find aspirin useful, be sure your physician knows how often you take it and the dose you use.

Acetaminophen [Tylenol and many others] is a medication that has many of the same treatment effects as aspirin but is technically in a separate class. Like aspirin, it is over-the-counter and can be helpful with many symptoms. Most patients know how much response they can get from acetaminophen. Do not exceed the recommended dosage, because this can cause liver damage in some people.

In the beginning of treatment, it is helpful to establish a regimen with a medication such as aspirin or acetaminophen to monitor the baseline response. From this baseline it becomes possible to judge responses with future medication attempts. It is also useful to assess just how much benefit, if any, can be gained from the simple medications. If judicious use of aspirin or acetaminophen will cause only a 10 percent reduction in symptom severity, at least it is better than nothing. The patient with CFIDS needs all the relief available and should not throw away a 10 percent improvement as long as it is safe.

Nonsteroidal Anti-inflammatory Drugs (NSAIDs)

There are a host of medications in this class, generally used for the treatment of pain and arthritis. Ibuprofen [Advil, Motrin, Nuprin], tolmetin [Tolectin], naproxen [Naprosyn], naproxen sodium [Anaprox], diflunisal [Dolobid], piroxicam [Feldene], meclofenamate [Meclomen], ketorolac [Toradol], and others are all variations on a theme and may be tried if aspirin or acetaminophen is not helpful. Some patients may benefit more from one agent in this class than from another, so a trial of different NSAIDs is possible. As with aspirin, abdominal pain and bleeding is a concern and should be monitored carefully by the primary care physician. The threat of intestinal bleeding is greater if these drugs are used in addition to aspirin.

Antihistamines

Patients with CFIDS may have worsening of allergies and upper airway congestion, and treatment with antihistamines may be useful. Because of the sedative effect of diphenhydramine [Benedryl and many others], this medication may be taken at bedtime and can even help treat the sleep disorder. However, it loses its effectiveness with continuous use past one or two weeks and so should be used only intermittently. Antihistamines are over-the-counter and may be tried cautiously. However, increase in daytime fatigue is a drawback to the use of most antihistamines. If allergy symptoms are to be treated with medications that have little or no sedation, terfenadine [Seldane] and others requiring a prescription may be tried.

Benzodiazepines

Tranquilizing agents, which require a prescription, may be useful in the overall treatment plan but should be used very carefully. Patients who experience agitation, anxiety, and panic attacks, despite marked fatigue, may be helped by these drugs. However, they may be habit forming; after long-term use, withdrawal from them can be extremely unpleasant, sometimes lasting for over six months. Therefore, the use of medications in this class, such as alprazolam [Xanax] and diazepam [Valium], should be intermittent and carefully monitored to prevent habituation.

Sleep disturbance has long been treated with drugs in the benzodiazepine class. But their value is greatest when the sleep disturbance is limited for a short period, such as a time of crisis. Chronic use reduces their effectiveness and makes getting to sleep without them more difficult. Some benzodiazepines, such as triazolam [Halcion], are short acting and can help initiate sleep, but should be avoided in CFIDS since the sleep disorder is a chronic condition. It should be used rarely, if at all.

My personal favorite for the sleep disorder in CFIDS is clonazepam [Klonopin], again used only in low doses and only intermittently. It is less habit forming than other members of the class and improves the quality of sleep. I would insist on "drug holidays" for any patient taking this medication. A number of researchers are looking at sleep studies in patients with CFIDS, and it will be interesting to look at the effects of clonazepam on sleep EEG and its value in improving symptoms.

Antidepressants

Patients are often distressed to hear that antidepressants are helpful in treating CFIDS because of the implication that depression is the cause of the illness. I do not believe that CFIDS is a form of depression, yet medications of this class may be helpful and are usually near the top of the list of medications I would try in the adult patient. The response to cyclic antidepressants is absolutely characteristic in CFIDS. If I were to choose a single diagnostic test for this illness, I would give a patient a standard dose of a cyclic antidepressant and observe the response. Patients with CFIDS are immobilized the next day, describing the effect as a hangover with severe fatigue. However, small doses of these medications may improve symptoms. The mechanism of action is unclear, and the improvement is unlikely to be due to lessening of depression. Among other things, cyclic antidepressants improve sleep quality and reduce pain. They require a prescription.

Doxepin [Sinequan and others], amitriptyline [Elavil, Endep, and others], desipramine [Norpramine and others], protriptyline [Vivactil], amoxapine [Asendin], nortriptyline [Pamelor], maprotiline [Ludiomil], and trimipramine maleate [Surmontil] are all drugs of this class and behave similarly. It has been suggested that clomipramine [Anafranil], also of this class, has a greater effect on pain relief than the others. Cyclobenzaprine [Flexeril] is also a cyclic antidepressant but is marketed as a muscle relaxant because of the prominence of these properties.

Patients with CFIDS who begin taking cyclic antidepressants should be told that they are likely to be sensitive to these medications. The initial dosage should be the lowest possible and then gradually raised to a point where the patient feels improvement without hangover. The improvement, if there is one, should be noted within a day or two rather than the several weeks expected in primary depression. If, however, depression is prominent in a patient with CFIDS, the medication trial should be carried out for at least a month before assessing the results.

My personal favorite is doxepin [Sinequan], because it has a sedative action in the first few hours. By using a low dose one half hour before bedtime, a patient with CFIDS may have help in going to sleep, improved sleep quality, and decreased fatigue during the day. For the patient unable to tolerate the lowest standard dose, doxepin comes in liquid form and the patient may experiment to find the most effective dose.

Other classes of antidepressants are also useful in CFIDS. Fluoxetine [Prozac], classified as a serotonin uptake inhibitor, has improved fatigue in many patients as long as the starting dose is very low. In normal doses, fluoxetine has the drawback of an unpleasant jittery feeling and worsening of insomnia. It should be taken in the morning at a low dose and gradually increased if tolerated. Formal studies about the use of fluoxetine in varying dosage schedules would be helpful for clinicians seeing patients with CFIDS. Sertraline [Zoloft] is a selective serotonin uptake inhibitor and may improve alertness and memory. Bupropion [Wellbutrin], of another antidepressant class, is known for its stimulant effects. CFIDS patients who have had seizures should avoid bupropion. Drugs classified as monoamine oxidase inhibitors, such as phenelzine [Nardil], have also been used in CFIDS, but they carry the risk of more serious side effects.

The Symptom Clusters

The patient must guide the physician in the treatment process. I always ask my patients what symptom or group of symptoms they would most like to be free from, since there are too many to blindly offer medications for all. A plan that will provide the greatest symptom relief with the least amount of risk should be formulated. I break the symptoms down into different categories and generally treat the categories in the following order.

Sleep Disturbance

Treating sleep disturbance first enables the physician to assess general responses to medication and the amount of variability of symptoms on a day-to-day basis. Try to assess how much fatigue is related to sleep disturbance. If the sleep disturbance is severe, an attempt should be made to improve sleep before trying to approach fatigue directly, because the medications may be quite different.

There are several options here. Sleep hygiene techniques are very important, with care to reset sleep phases. A sleep lab evaluation can be useful to treat concomitant conditions, such as sleep apnea. Antihistamines may be used on occasion, but the effect quickly vanishes on repeated use. Short-acting benzodiazepines will initiate sleep but are not helpful when you wake at 2 A.M. and cannot return to sleep. A longer-acting benzodiazepine such as clonazepam is an improvement. As mentioned before, benzodiazepines are not good for repeated, long-term use. The next step would be to add a cyclic antidepressant to an intermittent benzodiazepine.

Pain

Sometimes CFIDS patients have severe pain that can disrupt sleep. If pain seems to be causing or even contributing to the sleep disturbance, try treating the pain first. This treatment would be the same as for any painful condition: aspirin, acetaminophen, nonsteroidal anti-inflammatory medications. For severe pain, injectable ketorolac [Toradol] is a possibility, even for home use. I avoid all narcotics except in the most dire emergencies. The pain of CFIDS is a chronic condition, and habituation to narcotics will only worsen an already uncomfortable situation.

Again, the cyclic antidepressants are helpful in pain control and may decrease headache, muscle pain, and joint pain. The guidelines for using cyclic antidepressants are the same here as in their use for sleep disturbance. Clomipramine [Anafranil] or cyclobenzaprine [Flexeril] may be the most effective for pain control.

Fatigue and Malaise

Unfortunately, this symptom group is the hardest to treat. After approaching the fatigue through improving sleep quality, the next measure usually involves some type of stimulant. However, insomnia may become worse, eliminating any chance of improvement.

There are widely varying responses to stimulants in patients with CFIDS, and any attempt to use them should be approached with caution. If a patient has marked adrenalin symptoms or insomnia, I would not even attempt a trial with stimulants. Until controlled trials are conducted, primary care physicians should probably not venture past fluoxetine [Prozac] or bupropion [Wellbutrin].

The fatigue of CFIDS exists in two discrete types: The more severe CFIDS patients have an agitated exhaustion, characterized by tremulousness, weakness, and insomnia. This type of fatigue will invariably be worsened by stimulants. The second type of fatigue is characterized by hypersomnia or simple tiredness, and stimulants may be effective here.

One stimulant, low-dose amantadine, has been used for many years to treat the fatigue of multiple sclerosis and other neurologic diseases. Amantadine at the MS doses (100 mg twice daily) cannot usually be tolerated in CFIDS and may precipitate a relapse. I start with 25 mg in liquid form once daily, and slowly and very cautiously increase. Amantadine does not create energy where there is none; it will not return life to normal. It should be used with this in mind, and can make certain parts of the day more productive and comfortable. In a way amantadine in CFIDS is like the use of coffee in healthy persons. After running around following a few cups in the morning, a person may crash in the early afternoon.

Depression

I think the most important treatment for depression associated with CFIDS is an understanding of the illness and the usual good overall outcome. Acceptance of the limitation, and the support of physicians, family, and friends are important. Acceptance can be improved with professional counseling, just as in any chronic illness. If the depression is secondary to chronic malaise and loss of activity, treatment with the antidepressants already mentioned at low doses is helpful. If the depression is more severe, then full doses may be tolerated.

Cognitive Disturbance

The first approach to the cognitive symptoms should be through the treatment of fatigue. However, the more severe the illness, the more severe the nonfatigue cognitive symptoms. Low-dose naltrexone [Trexan] is an experimental treatment that has met with some success, with improved cognitive function in individual cases. However, no adequate treatment trials have confirmed this observation.

Catecholamine (Adrenalin) Symptoms

The symptoms of rapid heartbeat, palpitations, chest pain, hyperventilation, and panic attacks result from too much adrenalin stimulation, similar to what occurs with caffeine. As with many other symptom groups in CFIDS, standard medications are useful here. The rapid heartbeat and palpitations (sensation of fluttering) are usually easily treated with drugs called beta blockers, such as propranolol [Inderal and others]. However, some worsening of fatigue may be noticed and care should be exercised not to lower blood pressure. Low doses of a beta blocker usually suffice and may even help in reducing headache.

Abdominal Pain

Most clinicians have had experience in treating irritable bowel syndrome, and the same medications are worth a try in CFIDS. However, only a rare CFIDS patient has continuous severe abdominal pain. Usually there are episodes of severe pain followed by relatively long periods of mild symptoms, such as bloating and gas. Therefore, treatment for the abdominal symptoms should be limited, and when symptoms improve the medications may be stopped. Since most physicians are familiar with these medications, a complex discussion is not offered here.

Headache

As in the treatment of chronic pain, standard medications used for many years may be helpful with headache. Aspirin, acetaminophen, or the nonsteroidal anti-inflammatory medications are useful, particularly with steady doses. Medications used in migraine may also be tried, and some of the newer beta blockers and calcium channel blockers. Again both cyclic antidepressants and fluoxetine may play a role. There is a huge body of experience in treating headache. Although this can be a difficult and unpleasant symptom in CFIDS, it is also likely to be improved somewhat with treatment.

Some patients with CFIDS have a particularly severe type of pressure headache located at the base of their skull, that characteristically lasts for days. Possibly these headaches are brought on by elevations in the pressure of the brain's fluid system, and treatment with acetazolamide [Diamox] can be considered. As with other medications, acetazolamide should be started at low doses and used with caution; the response may take several days. If there is any worsening of the neurologic symptoms—numbness, tingling sensations, neuralgic pain, or balance disturbance—this medicine should be discontinued.

Conclusion

In summary, many medications are useful for the treatment of CFIDS symptoms. But medications represent only a part of the overall treatment of this condition. As we have seen, activity limitation, life style adjustment, and common sense are essential to improvement. For the physician treating CFIDS, a delicate balance must be struck between art, medicine, understanding, and above all, compassion. For the patient, communication and feedback are necessary in forming a treatment program with your doctor that works best for you.

CHAPTER 13

What Does the Future Hold?

*C*hapter twelve discussed medications that are familiar to all primary care physicians. But in the search for medications effective in CFIDS, some unusual treatments have been attempted. Most of these medications have been explored because of specific ideas as to what is the cause of CFIDS, and thus experience is biased. None of the medications listed here is without controversy, and full placebo-controlled, double-blind trials are usually lacking. Moreover, as a further cautionary note, we know little about the possible risks and side effects of many of these medications.

*T*reatment Possibilities

Antibiotics

The role of antibiotics in CFIDS has been confusing and difficult for patient and researcher alike. Many patients believe for several reasons that antibiotics are bad, and I try to avoid antibiotics in people with this philosophy. Antibiotics may have a limited role in the treatment of CFIDS, however, and are certainly helpful with specific infections that may complicate the course.

Part of the controversy involves the risk that antibiotic usage may cause the overgrowth of the yeast candida, and that this agent, or a neurotoxin of this agent, causes CFIDS. The medical literature is weak on this hypothesis and generally has not been supportive.

Furthermore, for a large number of patients with CFIDS, the illness begins with an infection such as sinusitis, bronchitis, or throat infection. Most physicians prescribe antibiotics to treat these problems, and when the illness progresses to CFIDS, antibiotics are implicated. But the opposite argument can be made. Because CFIDS is associated with mild immunodeficiency, the first stages may be characterized by localized infections. Therefore, the process of the illness may require more frequent antibiotic usage, although this neither treats the underlying condition nor influences the long-term course.

Thus the question is whether antibiotics caused CFIDS or were used to treat infections caused by a process that had already begun. My personal belief is that antibiotics neither cause the illness nor prevent progression.

Even without specific localized infections, an argument can be made for antibiotic usage, although at present this argument is weak. In children, particularly, the gradual onset may be characterized by repeated infections. Independent of CFIDS, some pediatricians prescribe continuous antibiotics to suppress the occurrence of these infections and disrupt the cycles of recurrent illness. And I have placed some children with CFIDS on a six-month course of suppressive antibiotics for just this reason. In the long run, I have not noticed a marked overall difference in those children treated with suppressive antibiotics from those without. Only one small study in the medical literature supports the use of antibiotics in CFIDS (Salit 85). Clearly, much more work needs to be done in this area, but for now I would support the use of antibiotics for specific identified infections that may complicate the course of CFIDS.

Acyclovir [Zovirax]

In the 1980s, great excitement was generated by the use of acyclovir as an antiviral in the treatment of CFIDS. I think it is an example of a hypothesis influencing treatment outcome. The hypothesis was that a herpes virus, Epstein-Barr virus, or human herpes virus 6 was the cause of CFIDS. Because acyclovir is known to have an anti-herpes virus effect, it was a logical treatment choice and likely to improve, if not cure, the illness.

Unfortunately, the hypothesis turned out to be wrong. Neither the Epstein-Barr virus nor HHV-6 is the cause of CFIDS, and acyclovir does not seem to have much of an effect in improving symptoms (Behan 88a; Straus et al. 88). However, some patients say that they feel better when they are taking acyclovir. It is possible that because of the immunologic abnormalities, an increased burden is placed on the body by herpes group viruses in some patients. Therefore, treatment of these trigger agents may have a limited effect. Sometimes, persistent cold sores respond to acyclovir. But at the present time it does not appear to be a satisfactory solution to CFIDS.

Ampligen

Tremendous excitement and hope have been generated by early reports of Poly I–poly C [Ampligen] in the treatment of CFIDS. Reports have appeared in patient newsletters and conferences since 1990, and more detailed accounts are pending (Strayer 91; Cotton 91).

The first report of good treatment results came from a single patient treated by Dr. Dan Peterson, who, like other severely ill patients, had responded to no other treatment. This was followed by an informal trial of the drug in sixteen additional patients. Again, the results were very encouraging, with improvement to the degree that many of these patients were able to return to work. Yet despite the good results, it does not look as if any of this group has been cured. But when you consider that severely ill patients have almost no response to other medications, these results begin to look a little more miraculous.

A formal drug study was authorized by the Food and Drug Administration (FDA), and nearly one hundred very sick patients were treated in five separate sites in a well-designed double-blind, placebo-controlled trial. The results are again encouraging, with activity improvement, decreased symptom severity, and lack of any significant side effects in the treated patients.

Ampligen has not been approved by the FDA and so is not presently available. The next set of studies are scheduled, but FDA approval is a long and arduous process. If approved, Ampligen is likely to be a difficult and expensive treatment. It is administered intravenously several times a week for long periods of time, six months to a year. The optimum dosage schedule and length of treatment is totally unknown. Because it is not commercially available, the price of the drug is also unknown. An oral form of Ampligen is being contemplated but has not been tested.

There is a wide variety of feelings generated by the news of this drug, ranging from excitement to discouragement. Patient support groups are angry at the snail's pace of research in the drug approval process. Personally, I am enthusiastic about Ampligen. I believe that any drug that can improve the symptoms of severely ill CFIDS patients, particularly the cognitive symptoms, is likely to work well on the patient with more average severity CFIDS. However, trials on these patients have not yet been attempted, and only time will determine if this optimism is justified.

Gamma Globulin

Injectable gamma globulin is another medication with a long history in treating CFIDS. A blood product consisting of pooled antibody, it has many standard medical uses. Gamma globulin might be effective in the treatment of CFIDS for three reasons: (1) If the cause of CFIDS were a common virus, gamma globulin would have high concentrations of specific antibody that would be directed against this agent. (2) If a trigger agent that begins the process of CFIDS were a common virus, again specific antibody would be helpful. (3) Gamma globulin preparations are also known to have immunomodulatory effects in addition to the presence of antibody. It is possible that these effects would dampen the immune up-regulation characteristic of the illness.

The first study to examine the use of gamma globulin in CFIDS showed that 56 percent of patients receiving a monthly injection improved, while only 32 percent of those receiving placebo improved (DuBois 86). There are two studies examining high-dose intravenous gamma globulin, and they present conflicting results. One trial used very high doses and noted a 43 percent improvement, against a 12 percent improvement with placebo (Lloyd 90). The second study used lower doses and showed no significant response (Peterson 90).

The appropriate role of gamma globulin in the treatment of CFIDS is still not known. If used intravenously, it is very expensive, and most insurance companies will not pay for it. It does not cure the illness even in those who seem to improve, and if a beneficial effect is noted, it wears off within a month. However, it is generally safe if given by clinicians experienced with its use.

Steroids

Many patients I have seen in consultation have received a course of steroids at some time or other during the course of their illness, and nearly all have had no significant effect. But little concerning this subject has appeared in the medical literature (Behan 88a).

One interesting role for steroids is to examine the possibility of another illness. Several autoimmune diseases can closely resemble CFIDS, illnesses that frequently respond to steroid treatment. A rare patient with early dermatomyositis will not have marked weakness or elevated sedimentation rate, and muscle biopsy is necessary to make the diagnosis. In that patient a trial with steroids will show remarkable improvement. However, if the retroviral hypothesis of the cause of CFIDS turns out to be correct, steroid treatment has important theoretical drawbacks, as steroids may permit viral growth.

Immunomodulatory Drugs

The concept of immunomodulation is to alter or modify the immune response. For theoretical reasons, immunomodulatory agents may be attractive for patients with severe symptoms. But there are many problems, and I have never attempted these agents in a patient with CFIDS.

As will be discussed in later chapters, it is possible that the symptoms themselves are due to an activated immune response.

In an attempt by the body to search out and destroy some offending agent, substances are made that cause the symptoms experienced by patients with CFIDS. Theoretically, if you turn off this hyperimmune response, the symptoms will disappear. However, what will happen if this hyperimmune response is turned off or blunted is not known.

The biggest concern that I would have with the use of immunomodulatory drugs is the possibility of turning an unpleasant disease into a dangerous one. These agents have serious side effects, and with an immune system that is already compromised, we do not know the long-term effects. There are hypothetical reasons why this area should be explored in the future. However, it will take carefully controlled trials to examine these agents, and they should not be tried haphazardly.

Stimulants

There have been no satisfactory trials with stimulants such as amphetamines, or pemoline [Cylert]. Moreover, to my knowledge, no researcher seems particularly excited about them, and it is unlikely that they will prove to be of much benefit.

Kutapressin

Kutapressin is a bovine liver extract used for many years as a nutritional supplement, much like an injection of B12. Again, little has appeared in the medical literature (Kaslow 89), and enthusiasm is limited to a few researchers.

One group, Drs. Steinbach and Herman, have used Kutapressin extensively and described their results in the Spring 1990 issue of *The CFIDS Chronicle*. Of 270 patients receiving at least ten injections, 75 percent improved and only 12 percent clearly failed to have a good treatment response. Only one patient had an adverse drug reaction. There are interesting theories as to whom Kutapressin may be of value to, but a large double-blind study is clearly needed before claims can be made.

Magnesium

As mentioned in the chapter on laboratory studies, red blood cell magnesium was found to be decreased in patients with CFIDS, and treatment with injections of 1 gram of magnesium sulphate improved symptoms (Cox 91a). Of the fifteen patients treated in the study, twelve improved, where as only three of seventeen on placebo were better. It was an exciting article, and numerous researchers tried magnesium on their own patients.

However, the follow-up studies have not been as exciting (Gantz 91; Clague 92; Durlach 92; Howard 92). It has been suggested that, because magnesium is a painful injection, patients were able to distinguish who was receiving the placebo and this could have influenced the results. But it remains a possibility, and until further confirmatory studies are done, I would concur with Dr. Gantz, who said, "Avoid treatment with intramuscular magnesium sulphate unless a deficiency can be demonstrated" (Gantz 91).

Evening Primrose Oil

In an article in 1988, treatment with Efamol, or Evening Primrose Oil, was noted to improve symptoms in a group of patients with CFIDS (Behan 88a; Behan 90). In the study, 84 percent of CFIDS patients had improved symptoms, compared to only 24 percent with placebo. If this turns out to be correct, it has important implications for understanding the mechanism of disease as well as for treatment.

Co-Enzyme Q10

This naturally occurring compound is sold as a nutritional supplement and does not require a prescription. Again, no studies have been published in the medical literature concerning its use, but it is common to hear a patient say that a modest improvement occurred with its use. I am not aware of any side effects.

Vitamin C

Numerous researchers have attempted infusions with vitamin C, although the medical literature is sparse (Ali 91). If it really works, it would be a great treatment because it is inexpensive and safe. Adequate trials need to be done to end years of speculation; without some consistent medical evidence of efficacy, insurance companies will not pay for its use as a symptomatic treatment.

Vitamin B12

For many years physicians would prescribe a shot of B12 for people who were not feeling up to par. In the 1950s, this practice began to disappear because medical studies had not proved any benefit. Giving B12 became a sign of archaic medicine, and the modern physician wanted to distance himself or herself from the old-style clinician.

Yet the old-style clinician may have observed a real effect. Certainly there is no B12 deficiency state present in CFIDS. Measurement of B12 levels is always normal, and treatment with B12 is not to replace a deficiency, as in pernicious anemia. Yet the doses that are talked about in CFIDS are not those for vitamin replacement; they are the doses used for a drug effect. B12 has numerous roles in the body, and it is possible that at high doses it may improve symptoms. Like vitamin C, it is well known, inexpensive, and safe. I have used it and have limited enthusiasm for it.

Anticandida Medications

Several researchers have presented information at patient conferences suggesting the effectiveness of diets and medications designed to eradicate the yeast candida. I do not have experience with this treatment, and there have been no adequate treatment trials to assess its efficacy. Because the treatment takes many months, and many patients with mild or moderate CFIDS have spontaneous improvement, it is necessary to see if these treatments really affect the course of the illness or reflect the passage of time.

Other Nutritional Supplements

In general, I am not qualified to discuss nutritional supplements. Articles concerning nutritional treatments have not been published in the standard medical literature, and rigorous trials are expensive and difficult to conduct. I would like to see greater openness on the part of practicing physicians to examining the subject, along with more evidence on the part of advocates of nutritional therapies. A newsletter describing therapies of this type, *Health Watch*, is available at 1187 Coast Village Road, #1-280, Santa Barbara, California, 93108.

Conclusion

I hope that by the time this book is published there will be numerous, proven, effective treatments available to patients with CFIDS, perhaps even treatments that can cure the underlying cause of the disorder. For this to occur, several things are needed. The most important is an increase in research interest in the illness. This interest is usually stimulated by research grant money, almost nonexistent in 1993. The cause of the illness, as well as the mechanism of symptoms, must be established. Treatment should be rational and based on well-conducted treatment trials. CFIDS needs to be taken seriously by the medical community and must move into the standard arena of medical research for true progress to be made.

PART 5

The Search for a Cause

CHAPTER 14

The Historical Perspective

*B*efore we can launch into new and promising research and theories that are being developed to find the cause and, ultimately, the cure for CFIDS, it is important to know the history of the illness. As with nearly every topic concerning this illness, the question of whether CFIDS is a new or an old disease has been debated. Those researchers arguing that CFIDS is an old illness point to descriptions dating back several hundred years to illnesses such as febricula or neurasthenia. Those arguing that CFIDS is new state that no illness this dramatic and this common could have been missed by the excellent clinicians of the past. But the question has no easy answers.

It is possible that CFIDS has been present for centuries but was never well recognized because of the more immediate concern for diseases such as smallpox and plague. Clinical descriptions of the past are hard for us to recognize today because of the archaic language used and changes in basic concepts of disease. Yet complex illnesses such as rheumatic fever have been well recognized.

*C*FIDS *Epidemics*

In the past few decades, there have been numerous outbreaks bearing a resemblance to CFIDS, and more than forty have been described in the medical literature. The outbreaks are usually named for the location in which they occur, and have been given little attention, perhaps because of the assumption that whatever had caused an outbreak was an isolated event. Descriptions vary in completeness and the emphasis varies from author to author; it is hard to make comparisons between them because outbreaks tend to be described in the terms of the particular specialty or bias of the discoverer.

The literature has emphasized epidemics, because the diagnosis of a complex collection of symptoms as a specific illness is easier when large numbers of cases are involved. Following are brief descriptions of some of the more well known epidemics, with an emphasis on certain points that are consistent within them. One case, that of Lyndonville, New York, is examined in more depth.

Los Angeles, 1934

Perhaps the first outbreak to give us good insight into CFIDS occurred in Los Angeles in 1934 among personnel at the Los Angeles County General Hospital. It was estimated that over 10 percent of the hospital staff—nearly two hundred people—became ill. This outbreak, like many others assumed now to be CFIDS, involved medical personnel and has led to an assumption that doctors, nurses, and other health care workers are at high risk. It remains to be seen if this is true, as medical care facilities such as hospitals or clinics are more likely to notice outbreaks when they occur. The spread of this illness at Los Angeles County General Hospital was assumed to be from personal contact between cases.

The outbreak coincided with and was assumed to be part of an epidemic of poliomyelitis. There were several differences, however, the most important of which was that despite weakness, patients did not develop the classic paralysis of polio. Moreover, the degree of muscle tenderness and generalized fatigue was greater than that seen in polio. Other differences became apparent as well, and the illness at Los Angeles County General Hospital was considered separate and called neuromyasthenia. In the clinical description, the prominence of vasomotor symptoms was emphasized, implying involvement of the autonomic nervous system. There were prolonged absences from work in the staff affected by this disease, and 55 percent were still unable to work six months after becoming ill. Follow-up studies indicated that recurrences of symptoms were prominent many years after the illness.

But the association with and similarity to poliomyelitis spurred beliefs that CFIDS might be due to a related or similar virus, an atypical polio virus. Another line of speculation was that the illness resulted from an unusual immunological reaction to an infection with the known polio viruses. Several other outbreaks of CFIDS have been linked to poliomyelitis in the past. This is not surprising and may be due both to similarities in the nature of the symptoms and to the tremendous concern about polio between 1930 and 1960.

Iceland, 1948

An epidemic, again suggestive of poliomyelitis, was reported in more than one thousand people in northern Iceland in 1948. Most of the cases occurred in and around the town of Akureyri, hence the names Akureyri disease and Iceland disease. There were three cases of classic polio with severe paralysis at the onset of the epidemic, but as in the Los Angeles outbreak, the following cases did not appear to be polio. There was, however, an outbreak of type 1 poliomyelitis present on Iceland at the time of this epidemic. Moreover, the areas where Iceland disease was prominent were spared from the polio epidemic. The patients affected with Iceland disease did not have antibodies to the three types of poliovirus, but when they were later immunized their antibody responses suggested a previous exposure to polio. In summary, the agent responsible for Iceland disease was not classic poliovirus, but it prevented subsequent development of the disease. This evidence suggests a close relationship with poliovirus, a feature that needs to be explained in any theory of CFIDS suggesting that Iceland disease is the same illness.

While all age ranges were affected, the outbreak was particularly intense among high-school children. It was rare in young children and in the elderly. Overall, 5 percent of the male population and

8 percent of the female population contracted the disease. The common symptoms were fatigue, malaise, emotional instability, muscle tenderness, and, of course, the protracted length of the illness. The epidemic appeared to be caused by an infectious agent with person-to-person spread and a short incubation period.

Comprehensive, detailed studies were carried out to determine the cause of this outbreak. Studies routinely done for poliomyelitis, as well as animal studies searching for new or related agents, were unrewarding. There were no deaths reported, but follow-up studies showed prominent disability and the presence of abnormal neurologic signs in many of the patients.

Adelaide, Australia, 1949

In the summer of 1949 another large outbreak was observed on the south coast of Australia. More than eight hundred cases of CFIDS were recorded during an outbreak of typical poliomyelitis, the differentiation being due to clinical features and normal spinal fluid. It again appeared that whatever was causing CFIDS inhibited the spread of polio or changed the course of the illness. During the investigations for a poliomyelitis-like agent in this outbreak, an agent was transmitted to monkeys that caused abnormalities in nerve preparations. However, further isolation of an infectious agent was unrewarding. It is of interest that this epidemic records a more equal male-female ratio, a feature that is slightly different from other outbreaks.

New York State, 1950

In Upstate New York an outbreak occurred in thirty-three patients, and similarities to "Iceland disease" were recognized at the time. The illness was termed "abortive poliomyelitis," and detailed studies were carried out on seventeen patients. The majority of patients studied had a gradual or insidious onset rather than the abrupt onset more frequently seen. In other respects the fatigue, muscle aching, neurologic complaints, and other symptoms were similar to those described in the Iceland outbreak. Eighteen months after the onset of symptoms, all patients continued to have fatigue and weakness, but none had wasting as is seen in polio. There have been two other recorded instances of outbreaks recorded in Upstate New York prior to the outbreak in Lyndon-ville in 1985.

Washington, D.C., 1953

An intense epidemic of an illness suggestive of CFIDS occurred near Washington, D.C., in 1953 in a psychiatric hospital. The out-break was studied in detail, again because the initial assumption was that the cause was paralytic poliomyelitis. Of the two hundred personnel at the hospital, fifty became ill, an attack rate of 25 per-cent; and half of those affected had paresis, or marked muscle weakness and pain. Again the typical findings of poliomyelitis were lacking.

There were two discrete parts to this epidemic, the majority of cases being among student nurses. Detailed epidemiologic studies led to the assumption that the cause was an infectious agent and that the incubation period was less than one week.

Royal Free Hospital, London, 1955

Perhaps one of the most important and controversial outbreaks occurred in 1955 in London's Royal Free Hospital. It is interesting to observe the parallels between this well-described outbreak and the perception of CFIDS in the United States thirty-five years later. The organic / psychosomatic arguments are virtually identical. So little has changed in thirty-five years.

The outbreak began when a physician and nurse were admitted to a ward of the Royal Free Hospital with an unusual illness in the early summer of 1955. This was followed by the same illness affecting more than seventy hospital personnel in the next few weeks. Overall, 292 staff members developed the symptoms, which became known as Royal Free disease, and the hospital was closed for four months. The early symptoms were malaise, fatigue, headache, and sore throat. Abdominal discomfort, diarrhea, muscle pain, bladder problems, dizziness, and weakness were prominent symptoms.

Numerous abnormalities were documented on physical examination of the patients in the early phases of the illness. Liver enlargement was found in 8.5 percent of the acute onset cases, and 34 percent of the patients had cranial nerve palsies, a higher incidence of this neurologic finding than in other epidemics. Lymph node enlargement was present in almost all patients, as well as tenderness in the liver and spleen areas. It was assumed that the illness was infectious and spread by personal contact, but only twelve inpatients of the hospital developed the illness. Numerous detailed attempts to find the cause of the illness were unsuccessful.

Perhaps the most remarkable aspect of the Royal Free epidemic was what occurred several years after the outbreak, when the case records were reviewed by consultants who had not seen or examined the patients. These consultants concluded that the epidemic was caused by mass hysteria, not an organic disease process. They cited the prominent emotional symptoms of the patients, the lack of deaths, and the improvement of symptoms over time. This official conclusion received wide press coverage and began the divisive and destructive debate over the nature of CFIDS that has continued to the present. Royal Free disease was the birth of the organic / psychosomatic argument.

Great Ormond Street, London, 1974

In 1974, the debate concerning Royal Free had barely died down when a similar outbreak occurred in the Hospital for Sick Children of Great Ormond Street in London. One hundred fifty staff members of the hospital became ill, an attack rate of 8 percent. The symptoms appeared to be the same as the illness described at the Royal Free Hospital, and this time the investigators were careful to look for the signs of mass hysteria at the time of their investigation. Their studies emphasized the numerous, although subtle, physical examination and laboratory findings, and they concluded that the illness could not be caused by hysteria. Once again, detailed studies for an infectious agent were unrewarding. This outbreak served to reinflame the Royal Free argument.

Ayrshire, Scotland, 1980

In the past fifteen years, the emphasis in Great Britain on myalgic encephalomyelitis (CFIDS) has revolved around the Coxsackie B virus. This dates to an outbreak occurring over a two-year span in Scotland. In these patients chest pain and cardiac symptoms were prominent, and as the Coxsackie virus is known to infect cardiac muscle, it became a logical suspect. Furthermore, the Coxsackie virus is a relative of poliomyelitis; both are members of the enterovirus family. In these studies it was noticed that 82 percent of the twenty-two patients studied had elevated antibody levels to the Coxsackie B virus. Numerous other studies have examined this relationship, and elevated antibody levels to Coxsackie have been found in other clusters. Any theory of the cause of CFIDS must explain these Coxsackie antibody findings.

Lake Tahoe, 1985

In the United States, interest in CFIDS was stimulated primarily by an outbreak in Lake Tahoe involving more than two hundred cases studied originally by Drs. Paul Cheney and Dan Peterson. At the time of this outbreak, papers had been published concerning persistence of the Epstein-Barr virus (EBV) in what was then called chronic Epstein-Barr virus disease. The EBV levels were measured in the Lake Tahoe patients and found to be elevated in up to one-third. Numerous other laboratory abnormalities were seen in these patients, and the outbreak was eventually studied by the Centers for Disease Control. Doubt was subsequently and legitimately raised about the role of EBV as the cause of the illness, but unfortunately this was interpreted to mean that there was doubt about the reality of the illness as well.

In March 1988 a consensus report sponsored by the Centers for Disease Control and authored by seventeen distinguished scientists was published in the *Annals of Internal Medicine*. In this report, specific guidelines were established for the diagnosis of the illness, and the name "chronic fatigue syndrome" (CFS) was suggested. CFIDS now officially existed in America and was a legitimate area of research (Holmes 88).

Lyndonville, New York, 1985: Anatomy of an Epidemic

The majority of patients who develop CFIDS are not known to be associated with a recognized outbreak or epidemic. These patients are considered sporadic or endemic cases, a term implying an infectious agent smoldering in a community and occasionally causing disease. Yet there have been numerous reports of clusters, as we have just discussed. The presence of both epidemic and endemic cases has generated discussion and controversy. Is there a difference between sporadic CFIDS and epidemic CFIDS? Do more epidemics occur but go unrecognized? Is there a difference between the symptoms of those affected in epidemics and those who are isolated cases? Some of these questions surface in the epidemic of Lyndonville, New York, in 1985. Let us examine this epidemic to see how the illness appeared in, and affected, a single community.

Lyndonville is a village of roughly seven hundred persons located on the southern shore of Lake Ontario, nearly halfway between the cities of Rochester and Buffalo, New York. It is a quiet, rural area, home of beautiful apple blossoms in the spring and brutal snowstorms in the winter. There is almost no industry, and farming is the main means of subsistence. The town is located in the middle of Orleans County, and while cases occurred throughout the county, the greatest concentration appeared to be in the village of Lyndonville. I had begun practicing medicine in the town in 1978.

Cases of what would later be called CFIDS had been occurring in Lyndonville for many years, although not recognized as a specific illness. In later studies of patients with this unique symptom complex, the date of onset extended back as far as 1960, as shown in Figure 14–1. It is not possible to ascertain if there were specific outbreaks in the past, but it would be likely. The patients

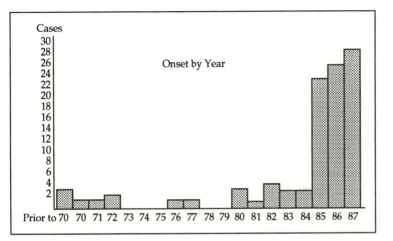

Figure 14–1: The year of onset of the first one hundred patients evaluated in the Lyndonville, New York, outbreak.

whose onset was prior to 1985 probably represented the minority of patients in past outbreaks who did not recover, since those patients who recovered spontaneously would remain unknown. Patients identified as having their onset from 1960 through 1984 would be considered to have endemic CFIDS, existing within the community but not connected to recognizable outbreaks.

In October 1985, eight children from two families became sick with an illness that superficially resembled mononucleosis. They had fever, enlarged and tender lymph nodes, exhaustion, sore throat, and abdominal pain, along with other symptoms. Two of the children had spleen enlargement. The illness differed from mononucleosis in subtle ways, however, and the blood tests for mono were negative. I assumed that these children had an acute viral illness.

Over the next month a number of other residents of Lyndonville, both children and adults, developed the same illness. Moreover, I recognized that a few patients I had been seeing for years had exactly the same pattern of symptoms, fatigue and flulike malaise being the most prominent. The eight children had not returned to normal health as would be expected with an ordinary viral illness, and some remained ill to the degree that they were unable to attend school or even leave the house. It was becoming clear that an unusual illness was present in the community, one that defied simple explanation.

My wife, Dr. Karen Bell, is an internist with subspecialty training in infectious diseases. In the early months of 1986 we developed diagnostic criteria for this illness by looking at the symptoms shared by the cases we had seen. The criteria were as follows: (1) symptoms for at least six months; (2) no evidence of other, known disease process; and (3) at least six of the eight major symptoms (fatigue, headache, abdominal pain, muscle pain, sore throat, lymph node pain, joint pain, and neurologic symptoms) and at least two of the minor symptoms (facial rash, pain on urination, eye pain or light sensitivity) (Bell and Bell 88).

She then designed a questionnaire for a case control study in an attempt to identify the cause of this illness. This questionnaire, reproduced in appendix 1, appears to be sensitive in identifying patients likely to have CFIDS. By March 1986 many adults and twenty-one children had been diagnosed with what we were calling Lyndonville chronic mononucleosis. It was decided to perform the case control study only on children.

Forty-two healthy children were matched by age and sex to the twenty-one cases identified, and all completed an extensive evaluation of potential factors. The prevalence rate among schoolchildren in the Lyndonville school system was found to be 2.7 percent, with an attack rate of 1.5 per 1,000 in 1984; 8 per 1,000 in 1985; 4 per 1,000 in 1986; and projected 6 per 1,000 in 1987. Three factors separated the children with CFIDS from healthy children in the community: (1) a medical history of allergies and/or asthma; (2) other family members with the same pattern of symptoms; and (3) a history of drinking unpasteurized milk. The results of this study were presented at the 1988 annual meeting of the Society for Epidemiologic Research (Bell 91).

The finding of raw-milk ingestion has been a puzzle ever since. Cultures of the milk in the surrounding areas revealed the usual bacteria known to cause human illness. In the first one hundred patients we evaluated, 83 percent had consumed raw or unpasteurized milk prior to developing CFIDS.

In a study to look more closely at a possible association between unpasteurized milk and the unusual illness, we evaluated two groups of people. The first group was 104 adults from a dairy goat growers association, 96 percent of whom drank unpasteurized milk frequently. The second group was composed of 178 adults who worked for an urban public health department. Because of their occupation and residence in an urban area, it surprised us that 25.3 percent had consumed raw milk at least on one occasion, and 16.9 percent had drunk it more than five times.

In the dairy goat growers association, 8 percent had at least eight symptoms of CFIDS and 23 percent had at least five symptoms, all of whom were raw-milk drinkers. In the control population only 2 percent were positive for eight symptoms, but 75 percent of those with symptoms drank raw milk. A further 11.2 percent had five symptoms of CFIDS, and again half of these were raw-milk drinkers. This study suggests a possible relationship between drinking unpasteurized milk and the symptoms of CFIDS. We found that several patients with a negative history of raw-milk consumption had been drinking it regularly at friends' houses without being aware that it was unpasteurized. However, it goes without saying that many people with CFIDS have never had unpasteurized milk. At the present time it is impossible to draw any conclusions from this study, which has not been repeated or confirmed.

The possible association with unpasteurized milk has been an enigma. If such an association exists, it may be due to a subclinical infection with a bacteria such as Yersinia enterocolitica that acted as a trigger for CFIDS, initiating the process. We have no evidence suggesting that Yersinia or any other milk-born bacteria is the cause of CFIDS. An alternative explanation might be that some other factor, such as a virus, pesticide, or toxin, may be initiating the response. These thoughts, however, remain entirely speculative.

In 1986, the histories of the first one hundred patients diagnosed as having CFIDS were evaluated, almost all of whom were from Orleans County. The majority (58 percent) were female. The average age was 27 years, and the average duration of illness was

40.5 months. The majority, 72 percent, had an acute onset of illness; the remaining 28 percent had a gradual onset. A separate study done at a later time showed no difference in the pattern or number of symptoms between those with acute onset and those with gradual or insidious onset. Allergies prior to becoming ill were present in 58 percent, asthma in 22 percent, and 16 percent had traveled outside of North America. Studies of socioeconomic status, divorce rates prior to developing CFIDS, and recognized mental illness showed no associations.

When questioned about what was the most severe and debilitating symptom, 49 percent said exhaustion, fatigue, or malaise. Headache was the worst symptom in 13 percent, cognitive disturbance in 7 percent, muscle pain in 7 percent, recurrent sore throat in 6 percent, lymph node pain in 5 percent, joint pain in 3 percent, and other symptoms in 5 percent. All patients had severe fatigue, and although it was the worst symptom in only half of the patients, all patients identified it as one of the three worst symptoms. The presence of symptoms in this group of one hundred patients are as follows:

Fatigue	100%
Neurologic	97%
Muscle pain	97%
Headache	95%
Eye pain or light sensitivity	94%
Recurrent sore throat	94%
Abdominal pain	92%
Lymph node pain	85%
Joint pain	80%
Flushing skin rash	74%
Recurrent fever	46%
Night sweats	46%
Chills	27%
Shortness of breath	14%
Palpitations	8%
Painful urination	6%

Physical examination of these patients was remarkably consistent. Lymph node tenderness was noted in 84 percent. The lymph nodes were not enlarged, however; only 2 percent had significant adenopathy. In retrospect, it is difficult to say whether muscle or lymph node tenderness was the more prominent. The majority of patients (60 percent) had significant muscle pain in sites away from lymph nodes. Abdominal pain was also common, being present in the right upper quadrant of the abdomen in 61 percent, left upper quadrant in 53 percent, and midabdomen in 58 percent. Rash could be seen in only 29 percent.

In those patients with a sudden onset of symptoms, more people developed CFIDS during the autumn months, but not to the degree of significance. My interpretation of this tendency is that a trigger infection caused the sudden onset of the CFIDS process, and these trigger infections are more likely to occur in the autumn or early winter. However, once again, alternative explanations are possible.

By 1990 the outbreak of CFIDS that affected Lyndonville, New York, had largely abated. Many patients had recovered completely, and the majority of the remainder are doing well, with near normal activity despite ongoing symptoms. A few patients remain housebound and totally disabled. In those patients diagnosed between 1985 and 1988, no other significant illness has been diagnosed that would cast doubt on the diagnosis of CFIDS. There are now two or three new cases every six months, which likely represents a return to the endemic level existing prior to 1984.

I believe that many outbreaks like that in Lyndonville have occurred across the country but have gone unrecognized. I have seen patients from different areas who have told me of clusters they are aware of. Endemic and epidemic CFIDS probably represent the same illness, perhaps modified by differing trigger factors. Although some worthwhile studies have emerged from the Lyndonville outbreak, the importance of the outbreak was overlooked for many years. It is unfortunate that so many research opportunities were lost.

Conclusion

A review of the medical literature on outbreaks reveals numerous subtle differences between them. However, considering the variety of countries involved and the changing local concerns from 1930 to 1990, these differences are minor. I believe that these epidemics were outbreaks of CFIDS.

The epidemics were intense with attack rates as high as 25 percent. They were "point epidemics"—they could stop as abruptly as they began. It was concluded in several outbreaks that the illness was caused by an infectious agent with an incubation period ranging from five days to two weeks. Casual personal contact was the likely means of transmission. The consequences of infection have been severe, with long-term disability common. In most outbreaks women were more commonly affected than men, but two outbreaks in military camps involving only men have been described. The disease has affected children as well as adults, and in communitywide epidemics up to 40 percent of cases were children. Several members of the same family could develop the illness at the same time, perhaps because of shared exposure to a common etiologic agent, shared genetic predisposition to the illness, or both.

It is unfortunate that the common or shared features of this illness are usually recognized only after the epidemic has passed. I hope that with increased awareness of CFIDS, outbreaks in the future will be quickly recognized and addressed. Complete and accurate documentation of the epidemiology and correlation with immunologic and other markers would be invaluable to our understanding of the illness.

CHAPTER 15

Theories and Research

*R*esearch on CFIDS has been conducted since 1938, when the first modern recognition took place. The association with polio epidemics was the first focus, and this association remains as much of an enigma now as it was fifty years ago. In an attempt to gain perspective, researchers began looking at different ideas, and the research has been rejuvenated with each fresh tack taken. But the illness remains a frustrating mystery—despite gains in many areas, the underlying cause is as hidden as before.

Or is it? In terms of knowing the cause, we are still in the dark. But researchers have now added many parts of the puzzle. We have approached the immune system abnormalities, and looked at different individual viruses that seem to be connected. We have described the neurologic and psychologic symptoms, and understand the nature of the disability with greater clarity. Yet doubt remains for some physicians even as to the existence of the illness, and it will probably persist until all pieces of this puzzle fit into a cohesive picture. Let us review the current state of CFIDS research to see how far along this puzzle has come.

One Disease or Many?

A basic and persistent question that has plagued researchers studying CFIDS is whether it is a single illness or a vague collection of many syndromes featuring fatigue. If it is a single syndrome, does it have one cause or many? There are probably as many answers to this question as there are researchers, and the variety demonstrates how little consensus exists on the fundamental nature of CFIDS. I have many friends among CFIDS researchers. Of two close friends, one believes that there are numerous illnesses, each with a different cause. The other believes this is a new illness with one single cause. You can imagine the fun we have at dinner after a conference.

It is a question that separates researchers into lumpers or splitters. Researchers who say that everyone with the CFIDS pattern of symptoms has the same illness are known as lumpers; they lump everything together as a single illness with a single cause. Those who say that there are many subgroups of patients, each with a different illness and cause, are the splitters; they subdivide CFIDS into numerous separate parts. There is evidence to support both points of view.

Lumpers and splitters can argue any illness. Of cancer a splitter would say there are numerous causes—chemicals, viruses, nuclear radiation; a lumper would say that all these causes are mere details that initiate cancerous growth by some common pathway. With respect to CFIDS, the dilemma can be represented by Figures 15-1 and 15-2.

The Splitter's Argument

Historically, the splitters have often been right. The atom, the basic unit of nature, turned out to have many discrete parts. Mental illness was not the result of bad humors but has numerous causes. At least five different agents can lead to what we know as infectious mononucleosis.

Let us examine some of the evidence of the multiple disease model. Perhaps the greatest hint toward the existence of multiple discrete illnesses making up the constellation of symptoms we call CFIDS is the variety of clinical patterns and the nonspecific nature of the symptoms. Because of a prominence of neurologic symptoms accompanying the fatigue, some CFIDS patients are diagnosed with atypical multiple sclerosis. Those with fatigue and prominent muscle pain have primary fibromyalgia. Fatigue plus severe headaches is called atypical migraine syndrome. Fatigue, palpitations, chest pain, and shortness of breath constitute mitral

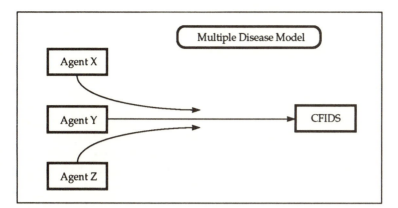

Figure 15–1: It is possible that several different factors, Agents X, Y, and Z, all cause the illness we call CFIDS.

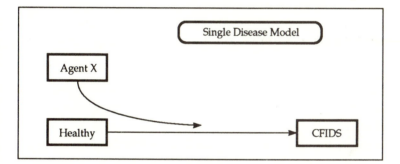

Figure 15–2: In this argument, CFIDS is a specific disease with a single cause.

valve prolapse syndrome. Some people have an acute and dramatic onset of symptoms of CFIDS, while others have a gradual and insidious onset. And on and on.

It is possible that these really are different illnesses that only superficially resemble each other with the passage of time. The epidemics in the different areas of the world have certain resemblances, but there are some interesting differences in details. Are the details real or due to observer bias? For example, the degree of muscle weakness seen in the Iceland epidemic appears to be greater than the weakness seen in the Lyndonville epidemic. The splitter would argue that the Iceland and Lyndonville illnesses are really completely different, caused by different agents, yet sharing a few common symptoms such as fatigue: separate disease states originating from separate causes.

The Lumper's Argument

Although I have tried to argue the case for the splitter, my bias, like that of several other researchers witnessing epidemics, is that of the lumper. Ten different illnesses could not have appeared in a small town by coincidence. More than 250 people developed the symptom pattern of CFIDS in Lyndonville, New York, and whatever caused this epidemic would have to be, in my opinion, a single event or illness. No more than a handful of patients had any other explanation for their symptoms.

Let us look a little more closely at some of the multiple disease model arguments. It is clearly true that numerous patterns of illness are seen in CFIDS, and these are especially prominent in the first six months. But several interesting points bring us back to the single disease model. Although patients have different degrees of severity of certain symptoms, the pattern is remarkably similar from patient to patient. Although a patient with atypical multiple sclerosis may initially look different from the one with primary fibromyalgia, closer examination reveals that the first patient also has muscle pain, although not to the same degree. In the first patient, the neurologic symptoms were of greater overall concern than the muscle aching and thus received greater attention. Both patients had the same pattern of symptoms, including the ones doctors don't frequently ask about: sore throat, lymph node tenderness, headache, concentration difficulties, abdominal pain, and night sweats.

In the Lyndonville outbreak, I witnessed different patterns of symptom severity within the same community. One patient might have severe neurologic symptoms whereas the next-door neighbor had severe joint symptoms. But both patients had the same overall pattern of symptoms, and it was my impression that they both had CFIDS. If so, it is unlikely that completely different causes of CFIDS existed in the same neighborhood. Indeed, even within some families I saw these variations in symptom pattern of those ill with what appeared to be the same illness.

Both types of onset—sudden acute onset and gradual onset—can be seen within families where more than one person was affected. In a study comparing the symptoms of those patients with each type of onset, two years after onset there was no significant difference between the symptoms of the two groups. That is to say, you could not predict the type of onset based on the symptoms after two years.

In reviewing the detailed descriptions of patients in earlier epidemics of CFIDS, or in discussing clinical details with a researcher who witnessed another epidemic, I clearly get a sense that although the basic symptom pattern is quite similar, there are some differences that do not appear to be explained by bias alone. My personal feeling is that there are different trigger events present in the different communities and that the minor variations seen are due to these differing trigger agents. For example, the epidemic in Los Angeles was closely correlated with poliovirus and seemed to have greater neurologic symptoms than the epidemic I witnessed. I think that this is a function of differing trigger agents, as shown in Figure 15-3.

A Compromise

It is possible to find a middle ground between the two arguments. After all, this may be no more than an exercise in semantics. We still talk of an atom being the basic unit of nature even though it is technically not true. AIDS is a single problem, but it is caused by two different viruses, HIV-1 and HIV-2, that are so similar we can almost consider them to be the same.

Furthermore, variation may be caused by individual host factors. One child with a strep throat will have less fever and more headache than another. Variation in host factors is a great unknown in CFIDS. But for practical purposes, I will continue to press the argument that CFIDS is a specific syndrome or collection of symptoms. I believe that it must have a single underlying cause. My only evidence for this statement is the lack of evidence. If

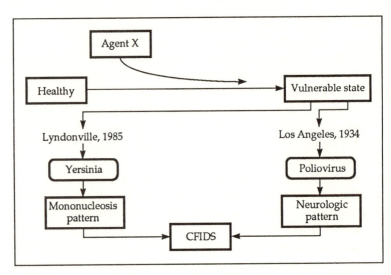

Figure 15–3: Minor differences in symptoms may be caused by different trigger agents, and not by a separate underlying cause.

there were fifty different causes for CFIDS, surely we would have found at least one by now. A splitter would call me a lumper with a clear tone of disgust. But these arguments are our way of having fun in medicine.

*T*he Spectrum of Theories

Most discussion around CFIDS has been among lumpers. There have been literally hundreds of theories attributing the symptoms of CFIDS to something or other, to one specific underlying cause. Splitters have not been interested in CFIDS. If it exists at all, it is most likely a name for an irrelevant collection of isolated, distinct illnesses. "Instead of an illness called CFIDS, we should study cancer, which causes fatigue, and sarcoidosis, which causes fatigue, and so on," the splitter would say.

The history of the theories put forward to explain this symptom complex has been fascinating, and an understanding of them will shed light on the nature of the syndrome. Obviously, any theory that ultimately proves true must be broad enough to explain the major points that have generated the numerous theories.

It goes without saying that every researcher has his or her own beliefs and biases. Although I have my own views as to the cause of the illness, I have great respect for all those with differing views. We live in an enormous and complex universe, and there is room for diversity. Furthermore, if we assume that there are more than one hundred theories about the cause of CFIDS, the statistical chance of my being in the correct camp is already less than 1 percent. I feel that in twenty years the details of this illness will be well known. What will have proven correct and what turned out to be just another wrong theory will be history.

The number of proposed causes for this strange and frightening disease is staggering. The number of symptoms of CFIDS is probably exceeded only by the number of theories proposed to explain them. This chapter will briefly outline a few of these theories and set the stage for a theory that I feel may encompass the mystifying details of CFIDS.

Any hypothetical cause, Agent X, needs impressive credentials to be a serious candidate as the cause of CFIDS. The fact that CFIDS has generated so much controversy is testimony to its complexity. Regardless of whether Agent X is a single causative agent or a combination of factors, there are numerous prerequisites. The ten conditions listed here are not universally accepted, but the majority of researchers would probably agree to at least most of them. Any hypothetical Agent X must be able to accomplish the following:

1. *It causes fatigue, exhaustion, and the other symptoms of this syndrome.* The symptoms are legion and form a unique pattern that defines CFIDS as a syndrome. The variety and pattern of symptoms are the most important of all prerequisites to fill. Many diseases have a few of the symptoms seen in CFIDS, but none have the whole pattern. Agent X must be able to cause all symptoms, either directly or indirectly.

2. *It affects children as well as adults but rarely affects children under the age of five.* Teenagers are frequent victims of the illness, but it occurs rarely under the age of five. It may be uncommon over age sixty-five as well. Any theory should be able to explain these curious details.

3. *It affects women more than men.* Among the adults affected, women have the illness more frequently than men. However, children have a more equal sex distribution.

4. *It causes both epidemics and sporadic cases.* Numerous epidemics of CFIDS have been recorded in the medical literature. However, there also appear to be isolated or sporadic cases not linked to any clearly recognized cluster.

5. *It is rarely, if ever, fatal.* This is an important prerequisite, and is linked to the lack of tissue or organ damage. The routine blood tests are normal, as are biopsy specimens from most sites. Whatever produces this illness causes no detectable damage to tissues, with the possible exception of minor hepatic and thyroid abnormalities.

6. *It causes immune dysfunction.* Agent X must not only be the cause of symptoms, but also be responsible for a confusing and complex dysregulation of the immune system. But Agent X does not cause severe immune deficiency.

7. *Onset of its symptoms may be either sudden or gradual.* Agent X must explain the different onset types. Any theory about Agent X also has to explain the variety of onset patterns and the vulnerable state that appears before onset in some patients.

8. *There is a spectrum of illness severity.* Some patients with CFIDS have an extremely severe illness with virtually no improvement over the years, whereas others have a mild form that is barely recognizable. In epidemics, which make the illness easier to diagnose, the entire range of symptom severity is seen.

9. *CFIDS occurs more commonly in patients with a history of allergy and/or asthma.* Any Agent X must be able to explain this finding.

10. *There is an increased incidence of CFIDS within families.* The increase of CFIDS among family members has been noted in many studies, and any comprehensive theory of the illness must explain this finding.

Persistent Infection with a Single Agent

This theory is the most straightforward, and I call it the "lumper's dream." Its appeal lies in its simplicity. It maintains that Agent X is a single agent, either virus, bacteria, or fungus, that by itself causes all the symptoms of CFIDS. The Epstein-Barr virus and some of the other possible agents were discussed earlier. These theories have been circulating for many years, and different candidate agents seem to come and go with the seasons. So far all have come up short.

Viruses are usually the first to be mentioned with this theory, and one name, "post-viral fatigue syndrome," directly names a viral agent as the cause. The first virus felt to be responsible was poliovirus, and many of the early epidemics appeared to coincide with epidemics of polio. Support for this theory came from some indirect studies and from evidence that patients with CFIDS have increased antibody levels to enteroviruses in general, of which polio and Coxsackie are family members. An unidentified close relative of the poliovirus has been suggested as the cause. In the United States attention focused on the Epstein-Barr virus and other members of the herpes virus class as the specific cause of CFIDS.

In Great Britain, Coxsackie B virus has been investigated as the possible cause for almost the same reasons we have been focusing on Epstein-Barr. The new human herpes virus, HHV-6, was also considered a likely candidate, and again the antibody levels appeared to be elevated. However, despite the interest in poliovirus, Coxsackie virus, Epstein-Barr virus, human herpes virus 6, and others, none of these agents can be consistently identified with patients who have CFIDS. Therefore, none of them fulfills the requirements as a single, underlying cause of CFIDS.

Thus, any theory involving common viruses as the sole etiologic agent has serious flaws. As discussed in chapter 7, the antibody levels to these viruses were noted to be elevated, which at first implied their being causative but subsequently was attributed to altered immune function.

While viruses are usually the first to be mentioned with the single agent theory of CFIDS, they are certainly not the only possible agents. Numerous nonviral agents can cause infections that share many of the symptoms of CFIDS. Notable among this group would be the organism that causes Lyme disease. Other nonviral candidates would include the bacteria that cause brucellosis or listeriosis, and the parasite that causes toxoplasmosis. However, these are well-known infections, and none fits the full description of CFIDS. Moreover, when these agents are looked for, the search is usually unrewarding.

It has been proposed that candida or possibly a toxin from candida is the cause of CFIDS. This theory postulates that candida, also called yeast, is the underlying Agent X because it is seen in increased frequency in patients. Candida is a ubiquitous organism that everyone carries. Infants develop thrush, a mouth infection characterized by white patches of yeast, also called oral candidiasis. However, with a normally functioning immune system, immunity rapidly develops, and there should be no further problems with candida except for an occasional vaginal infection in women, especially with antibiotics usage or diabetes.

Severe infections with candida are known to exist in AIDS because the immune system is not functioning properly. In CFIDS, up to 20 percent of patients may have oral candidiasis or give a history of a thick white coating on the tongue. As with many other potential Agent Xs, the question arises: Is the presence of this particular agent the cause of the disease or its consequence? With respect to candida, I believe that it is present in slightly increased quantities, probably due to the immune dysfunction of CFIDS. However, candida does not represent a serious threat as in more serious immune deficiency states. I believe that candida is present because of the illness and is not the cause of it.

One variation of the persistent infection theory, to be discussed in more detail later, is an infection with one of a class of agents known for chronic infections, the retrovirus. If a retroviral infection were the cause of CFIDS, the agent could not be one of the known human retroviruses, as these have not been found. The appeal is mostly theoretical at present, as retroviruses are known to infect both neurologic and immunologic tissues, causing neurologic symptoms, immune dysregulation, and chronic disease. The technology necessary to uncover retroviruses is in its infancy, and they may be the key to many unanswered questions.

Common End Pathway

The most widely accepted multiple agent theory involves a common end pathway that would provide a genetic mechanism for multiple different agents to cause the same immunologic reaction, thus resulting in the same illness. It is possible that agents such as the Epstein-Barr virus, human herpes virus 6, brucella, Coxsackie, and others, in patients that are genetically susceptible, may initiate an unusual immune state that may then cause the symptoms of CFIDS (Lloyd, Hickie and Wakefield 90).

In this theory each of those agents we have called trigger factors is a causative agent in its own right, and they do not usually cause CFIDS because of unknown genetic factors. That is, the genetic factors allow these agents to act differently in susceptible persons, thus causing a prolonged course of fatigue and other symptoms. Because of the unifying genetic factors, the end result is the same; they go through a common end pathway to produce a specific constellation of symptoms. In 1989 Hotchin presented evidence of multiple primary agents. The common end pathway theory is similar in concept to the trigger agents. In the former, however, the disease is a genetically susceptible immune system, whereas in the latter it would be an acquired defect in immune function.

One appealing aspect of the common end pathway theory is that we already know of examples in clinical medicine. Infectious mononucleosis is itself a common end pathway initiated by several different infectious agents. Reactive arthritis is the joint pain seen after bacterial and viral infections and is thought to be caused by a shared immunologic reaction to the various agents. But these known examples are different because they do not persist for as long as CFIDS, nor do they cause the amount of disability.

Camel's Back Theory

A variant of the common end pathway hypothesis is the camel's back theory. The principle behind this theory is that the body in general, and the immune system in particular, face numerous insults, and that after a certain degree of insult the whole system breaks down. Something occurs, either infection with the Epstein-Barr virus or immune damage from toxic exposures, that "breaks the camel's back," and the symptoms of CFIDS ensue as a nonspecific result of the damaged immunity. In this theory there is no single Agent X, but a whole host of agents causing damage to the immune system. When a critical amount of damage occurs, a state of dysfunction causes the symptoms.

Abnormal Response to Infection

There are illnesses known to be initiated by specific infections, yet the damage caused by these illnesses is from an abnormal immunologic response. Perhaps the best known is rheumatic fever, where an infection with the strep germ causes a serious disease of heart muscle. In rheumatic fever, the body makes antibodies to the strep germ, but because the strep germ looks like heart muscle to the immune system, it directly attacks the heart muscle as well as the bacteria. Such a process is called "infection stimulated autoimmunity."

As mentioned in the chapter on immunology, autoimmunity is a regular feature of CFIDS. Could there be an autoantibody, created by an initial infection, that is directed toward some body tissue that causes the symptom complex of CFIDS (Behan 88a)? If so, this theory would be a variation of the common end pathway theory, as numerous initiating events would set it off.

But there are many drawbacks to this theory. While autoimmunity may be present in CFIDS, it is extremely mild, almost trivial. Biopsy samples do not show the characteristic inflammatory changes often seen in autoimmunity, and the sed rate, a marker for inflammation, is low. Furthermore, the symptoms are not confined to a single peripheral organ system as in autoimmune disease. Back to the drawing boards.

Subacute Thyroiditis or Hypothyroidism

One organ that is occasionally involved in an autoimmune process in CFIDS is the thyroid gland. It is possible that abnormal functioning of the thyroid gland may actually cause CFIDS (Weinstein 87). The primary reason for this hypothesis is that many of the symptoms of CFIDS can be explained by a decreased metabolic rate, a prominent aspect of hypothyroidism. The low basal temperature, sluggishness, hair loss, and weight gain are also suggestive symptoms.

A few CFIDS patients develop abnormal thyroid function during the course of the illness; they develop hypothyroidism, or autoimmune inflammation of the thyroid gland leading to low thyroid hormone production. But the majority of patients have normal thyroid hormone levels. The argument here is that the thyroid hormone is not accomplishing its task—there is a functional hypothyroidism. An adequate level for healthy persons is not normal for the CFIDS patient. For example, it has been suggested that in illnesses with excess levels of cytokines (to be discussed in the next chapter), the function of thyroid hormone is blocked.

If this were the case, treatment with thyroid preparations might improve the symptoms. I would like to say that thyroid replacement is the solution to the problems of CFIDS. It would be a wonderful, safe, and simple treatment. Unfortunately, I have not found it to be effective.

Primary Emotional Disorder

Perhaps the most widely discussed theories are those that maintain that CFIDS is an emotional disorder, a form of mental illness. In these theories the common underlying theme is that an abnormal mental response causes the symptoms to appear.

At one extreme is the argument that CFIDS should not even be considered an illness, but rather a collection socially molded behaviors, "explanatory labels for a wide variety of functional somatic symptoms" (Abbey 91a). At the other extreme is the argument that "depression and other psychological abnormalities may be manifestations of the syndrome" (Holmes 91a). In an attempt to combine viral infection with persistence of symptoms, it has been argued that an initial viral infection leads to a period of inactivity in which deconditioning occurs. This is then followed by a vicious cycle of inactivity, depression, and deterioration of exercise tolerance leading to worsening of fatigue, muscle pain, and other symptoms (Wessely and Powell 89).

As this subject was discussed earlier, we will not dwell on it here. But the entire discussion of emotions and depression in CFIDS can be summed up nicely: "CFS by design resembles psychiatric diagnoses more than traditionally defined medical disorders because it represents descriptive phenomenology" (Krupp 91). That is to say, a psychiatric diagnosis is suggested whenever description replaces technological measurements.

Encephalitis

Inflammation of the brain is known as encephalitis. In the early descriptions of the Royal Free and other epidemics, the presence of neurologic symptoms and signs led investigators to believe that encephalitis was present, and the term "myalgic encephalomyelitis" has been used in Europe ever since. While many researchers maintain that there is no brain inflammation in CFIDS, it is an assumption never demonstrated. But if CFIDS is a form of encephalitis, it is different from those in the textbooks.

One way to look for brain inflammation is by examination of the spinal fluid. If excess numbers of white blood cells are seen, inflammation can be suspected. In CFIDS, both the spinal fluid protein and the white blood count are sometimes elevated, usually in the patient with more severe illness (Komaroff 88; Warner 89). Studies are increasingly demonstrating abnormalities within the brain, in its ability to regulate hormones (Demitrack, Dale et al. 91) to magnetic resonance abnormalities (Buchwald 92) to abnormal blood flow distribution (Douli 92).

In CFIDS there is a process in place that seems to decrease the brain's arousal (Grafman 91). That is, some process, whether infection, inflammation, or injury, is causing the brain to shut down, causing fatigue and other symptoms. The messenger chemicals of the brain are disturbed, and the pattern in CFIDS can resemble the brain after a period of drug abuse (Lehrer 88).

At present, the question is not so much whether the brain is involved in CFIDS, but exactly how and what is causing it. CFIDS does not look like most infectious encephalopathies, but we know of viral infections of the brain that do not show up in spinal fluid. The similarity between CFIDS and the fatigue following head trauma is another interesting area that deserves further study.

Primary Sleep Disorder

The argument that many of the symptoms of CFIDS are from lack of effective sleep is interesting and probably correct. As the sleep center is located in the brain, sleep is part of neurologic functioning, thus making this theory a variation of the encephalitis theory. Frequently I hear a patient say, "If only I could get a good night's sleep. . . ." Exhaustion without the ability to sleep is a frequent symptom, nearly as frequent as waking without feeling refreshed. In this theory, some primary disturbance of effective sleep results in the common symptoms of CFIDS.

It is interesting that we know so little about sleep. What does it do? What are dreams for? It is possible to visualize the symptoms of CFIDS for a day following an all-night poker game. Excessive stimulation and lack of sleep lead to exhaustion, achiness, a scratchy throat. In fact, one study of healthy students produced the muscle pain of fibromyalgia by depriving them of one stage of sleep (Moldofsky 89b).

Primary Immunologic Disorder

A primary disturbance of the immune system, creating excessive normal body chemicals known as cytokines, is a leading theory as the cause of the symptoms of CFIDS (Kibler 85; Tosato 85; Dwyer 88; Lloyd, Hickie and Wakefield 90). This theory satisfies most of the prerequisites for CFIDS and will be discussed in greater detail in the next chapter. Cytokines, natural chemicals produced in cells, serve to transmit messages or instructions between different types of cells. When produced in excess or given by injection, they cause the body little harm yet generate symptoms strikingly similar to those of CFIDS. In this theory, the underlying cause of CFIDS, Agent X, stimulates the production of cytokines, which in turn cause the symptoms of CFIDS. The Epstein-Barr virus and other agents would not be the cause of CFIDS, but are triggers for the increased production of cytokines.

Perhaps the most exciting development in the science of medicine in the past ten years has been the increased understanding of cytokines. We are beginning to understand the mechanics of what actually causes symptoms in illness. CFIDS has been said not to be real because of the commonplace nature of the symptoms and the lack of tissue damage. With CFIDS, we are witnessing another era in medicine: the boundaries of "real" and "psychosomatic" are changing.

Chronic Metabolic Myopathy

The mitochondria are the cellular organs responsible for conversion of foods to energy. Defects of mitochondria will profoundly affect the cell, resulting in decreased energy production and the resulting loss of cellular functions. Most diseases of mitochondria that have been studied in detail are recognized soon after birth and are fatal, because all mitochondria in all cells are affected. But mitochondrial disease would be very hard to detect even with modern technology if only a portion of the mitochondria in a given cell were defective. The metabolic myopathy theory suggests just that: there is a partial defect, perhaps acquired, in mitochondria that causes a decreased energy production and metabolic derangement of cells.

Limited mitochondrial studies in two small groups of patients with CFS showed no marked abnormalities (Byrne 87; Byrne 88).

However, more recent studies have shown a defect in mitochondrial metabolism (Kuratsone 92).

Prominent among symptoms of CFIDS is muscle pain and weakness, emphasized in the many epidemics, and by itself suggestive of a mitochondrial energy defect. Muscle pain, called myalgia, may be due to inflammation of the muscle by viral agents, and viral nuclear material has been found in muscle tissue (Archard 88). It is possible that this low-grade viral infection of muscles, known as a myopathy, causes abnormal oxygen utilization and metabolic abnormalities that lead to fatigue and other symptoms. This has been one of the leading theories in Great Britain where the study of Coxsackie viruses has been prominent.

In another early paper, 75 percent of fifty skeletal muscle biopsies showed scattered muscle fiber destruction, and bizarre tubular structures in mitochondria (Behan 88a). In a subsequent study by the same author, mitochondrial damage was noted in forty-five of sixty muscle biopsies (Behan 91). Ragged red fibers were found on one muscle biopsy sample, implying a defect in energy production. It is quite possible that mitochondrial defects are present and can be seen in muscle tissue that create decreased energy production. The brain is very sensitive to energy production. But because it cannot be studied directly, hints about energy production would have to be found in muscle tissue.

Abnormal Rheology (Red Blood Cell Disorder)

There have been disputed reports that an abnormality exists in the outer membrane of the red blood cells, and that this abnormality alters the shape of blood cells (Simpson 86; Simpson 89; Wakefield 87). This can be visualized on electron micrographs of the red blood cells that show abnormalities in shape (Mukherjee 87). If these membrane abnormalities exist, they would cause abnormal blood rheology, or flow mechanics. The abnormal rheology would alter circulation in small capillaries and prevent adequate oxygen from reaching the tissues. The lack of oxygen in turn could cause a buildup of metabolic products that in turn might cause fatigue and other symptoms.

I am interested in this theory, because there appears to be a mild elevation in the red blood cell breakdown products in many patients, and this could be caused by a membrane abnormality. A major factor against this theory is that people known to have marked red blood cell abnormalities (hemolytic anemia) do not show the same symptoms seen in CFIDS. In the next year or so there will probably be more evidence to either support or eliminate this theory.

Environmental Illness

Many of the symptoms of CFIDS are similar to symptoms seen in heavy metal and other types of environmental poisoning. This similarity suggests either that CFIDS may be caused by poisoning or that some of the same mechanisms may play a role in the production of symptoms. The mechanism of symptoms is from a toxic substance causing mitochondrial or other cellular damage by disrupting the normal pathways the body uses to generate energy. Arguments against this theory include the lack of evidence for heavy metal poisoning found in those patients in whom it has been searched for.

Putting It Together

While at first glance this list of theories seems disparate and unconnected, it is possible to generate a theory consistent with much of the known data. We may be seeing individual descriptions of the different parts of an elephant, each delicately described, that can be merged to form a unified whole.

As any patient with CFIDS will tell you, the problem is "not enough energy." It is possible that the primary defect of CFIDS is a defect of energy production, probably from a mitochondrial defect. Because the brain is so exquisitely sensitive to energy production, the effects are most noted in the brain, probably the midbrain, including the centers controlling arousal, hormones, and sleep. This defect in energy production is initiated by a viral infection, perhaps mediated by the production of cytokines. To propose a viral infection able to cause mitochondrial defects is to enter a gray area of medicine—but CFIDS researchers have long been accused of operating in gray areas. The cytokine theory is the subject of the next chapter.

CHAPTER 16

A Promising Theory

Perhaps the most exciting development in the study of CFIDS has been the cytokine theory of symptoms, which for the first time explained both the many seemingly unrelated symptoms and their bizarre pattern and therefore merits special attention. How could one disease produce such diverse symptoms as joint pain and memory loss? Depression and fever? Rash and fatigue? Sore throat and abdominal pain? Herein might lie the answer.

CFIDS and the Flu

Of course, the flu can cause all these symptoms and still allow a relatively normal physical exam. But the flu is of short duration, and after a few days of discomfort the symptoms vanish. Furthermore, CFIDS is not caused by the influenza virus. Mononucleosis has certain similarities, but also goes away after a relatively short period of time. We know that specific viruses cause the flu and mono, but how do they actually cause the symptoms? If these illnesses are similar to CFIDS, perhaps by looking at the mechanisms of how the symptoms are generated we could gain some insight into what produces the symptoms of CFIDS.

Oddly enough, the influenza virus does not cause the symptoms of the flu by itself. Our own body's immune response to the influenza virus does. Most people assume a simple cause-and-effect relationship, but flu symptoms are mediated by certain chemicals made during the body's immune response. Indirectly, of course, the influenza virus is responsible because it sets this immune process in motion, but the virus itself causes few physical symptoms. The actual symptoms of fever, headache, muscle aching, nausea, and malaise are caused by the immune activation stimulated by the influenza virus. The body chemicals produced when the immune system is activated are called cytokines, and they are normally generated in response to viral infections.

For example, on Tuesday afternoon someone with the flu coughs near you and directly transmits the influenza virus to you. You breathe in the virus particles, and they begin an infection in your upper respiratory tract. They invade cells of the throat and lungs and begin to replicate. But you feel well and have no symptoms on Tuesday, Wednesday, or Thursday, despite the fact that the virus is thriving in your body. The period when the virus is growing and you feel well is called the prodrome of the flu. Although you feel perfectly well, the virus is present in large quantities, and you can transmit the infection to others during this stage.

On Saturday afternoon, however, you develop fever, chills, muscle aching, and sore throat. You have nausea, diarrhea, and develop a terrible headache. You are exhausted and crawl into bed to sleep. You have the flu.

It was Saturday afternoon when the immune system realized that the body was under attack by the influenza virus. As it should, it launched a counterattack against the virus by mounting an immune response. And it was this immune counterattack that made you feel sick. Specifically, the production of cytokines was the first step in this immune response. Therefore, the influenza virus is only an indirect cause of the flu symptoms; the cytokines are the direct cause.

But the immune system works well. The cytokines that were produced on Saturday direct the actions of the subsequent immune responses, such as the activation of certain types of lymphocytes, the production of antibodies, and so on. After a couple of days these mechanisms take effect and the influenza virus is destroyed. With the situation under control, the suppressor mechanisms take over and the system begins to shut down. The cytokines are no longer produced and the symptoms abate. Specific memory lymphocytes are produced to guard against this particular strain of influenza virus causing another attack. After a week you feel well and return to work.

C*FIDS and Cytokines*

The cytokine theory of CFIDS is simple. In effect, it says that with the onset of CFIDS this same immune response is initiated, but instead of completing its job and shutting down in a week, the response continues indefinitely. Instead of the cytokines being produced in a short burst of one week, they are initiated and the immune system is activated but does not shut off. The immune system becomes chronically up-regulated.

The irony of this theory is that Agent X, the hypothetical underlying cause of CFIDS, causes virtually no symptoms. It merely initiates the process of immune system activation and then sits by while the cytokines cause the owner to be sick. Of course, it is possible that Agent X would be causing damage to the different organs of the body if this process were not going on.

Many clinical aspects of CFIDS support the cytokine theory. The symptoms usually occur with an acute flulike onset, and the symptoms persist. This hints that the same mechanism that causes flu symptoms may be persisting in CFIDS. Second, no evidence of tissue damage occurs in CFIDS. If there were direct viral or bacterial invasion of tissues, abnormal blood tests would develop, and these are not seen. If the symptoms were caused by the normal body process of immune system activation by the cytokines, abnormal blood tests would not be expected. Again the analogy with the flu holds: if a person is sick with the flu, the doctor can find little wrong on physical examination or routine blood tests.

The gradual onset of symptoms in CFIDS is intriguing. As mentioned, it is possible that the underlying cause of CFIDS, Agent X, produces few or no symptoms when first acquired. It is the stealth bomber of the viral world and quietly establishes itself in the host as an infection, much like the prodrome of the influenza virus. But after some time, months or years, the immune system gradually becomes aware of its presence and begins its search by producing the cytokines. The symptoms of CFIDS thus begin gradually. Another option is that a trigger infection, such as acute mononucleosis, sets off cytokine production, which remains in a state of chronic activation. Instead of the mononucleosis resolving as it should, the symptoms persist.

It is interesting that in cases of acute onset of CFIDS symptoms, careful questioning often discloses numerous minor symptoms that had appeared months beforehand—the vulnerable state. Does this vulnerable state represent the early, almost insignificant symptoms caused by Agent X?

Another detail that supports the belief that cytokines cause the symptoms of CFIDS is that the illness almost never occurs under the age of five and is relatively rare under the age of ten. When young children do get CFIDS, it is relatively mild and almost always of gradual onset. After puberty, however, the symptoms may be as severe as in adults. This pattern of illness in which the severity is age dependent suggests an immunologic mechanism for the symptoms, as younger children do not have a fixed immunologic reaction and are therefore more tolerant.

Research with cytokines also provides other interesting ties to CFIDS. For the past five years, there has been intense study of one cytokine, Interleukin-2, because it has been promising in the treatment of cancer. In some of these studies, Interleukin-2 (IL-2) is purified and injected into patients with cancer, where it stimulates the immune response, sometimes with dramatic effects in destroying malignant cells. The therapy is not without side effects. IL-2 virtually always produces certain symptoms, fatigue, exhaustion, and flulike malaise being among the most prominent. Patients treated with IL-2 develop muscle and joint pain, sleep disturbance, chills, nausea, vomiting, diarrhea, disorientation, apathy, cognitive abnormalities, and memory disturbances.

In some studies severe psychiatric side effects were seen with IL-2, and these effects are related to the dose given. When the treatment was withdrawn, the effects returned to baseline. In the cytokine theory of CFIDS, the argument over whether CFIDS symptoms are organic or psychiatric becomes meaningless. The psychiatric symptoms are organic.

Interferon is another cytokine known to cause many of the symptoms normally seen in CFIDS. Again, much of our knowledge about interferon comes from its use as a therapeutic agent in the treatment of many conditions, from infections to cancer. Interferon is also known to cause fatigue, exhaustion, fever, bone and muscle pain, and numerous neurologic symptoms. Decreased attention span, short-term memory problems, and depression are also prominent. Again, all of these are symptoms of CFIDS.

The study of cytokines is in its infancy. They are difficult to measure accurately, and much more work needs to be done before the presence of cytokines in patients with CFIDS proves that they are causing the symptoms. But this theory offers an explanation for many of the troubling details of this illness and can be tested in future research.

Cytokines and Agent X

The basis of the cytokine theory is that the normal immune mechanisms of the body, when activated, can cause the numerous symptoms seen in CFIDS. This theory is not about the identity of Agent X; it is about the mechanism of how symptoms are caused. The activation of the cytokines is presumably due to an underlying cause, Agent X.

This pattern of immune system activation suggests a system desperately trying to achieve something, possibly struggling against Agent X. Preliminary studies suggest that when a person comes down with CFIDS the immune system is activated, and produces cytokines, in much the same way as would happen with usual viral infections. However, in CFIDS this mechanism fails to shut down, either because it is unable to accomplish its task or because of damage to the system. The majority of the symptoms of CFIDS can be explained by immune system activation alone. And this is the mystery of CFIDS. Instead of Agent X causing symptoms and damage as we are used to seeing in medicine, the symptoms are caused by our own immune response. Skeptics thus say that there is no disease, by which they mean tissue damage by a pathologic agent, causing symptoms. And they may be right! The symptoms are due to our own hyperimmune reaction. But the obvious implication is that there is a reason for the immune system to react, to defend against Agent X, whatever it may be.

For years we have been looking for the invading organism and have been remarkably unsuccessful. We have pursued the reactivated viruses under the assumption that they are causing disease. Sometimes we note a trigger infection, which appears to set off the process, but by themselves neither the reactivated viruses nor the trigger infections can explain the range and persistence of symptoms.

Again the arguments of the skeptics can help us. The symptoms are "normal" symptoms, perhaps just a little more severe than usual. That is, there is nothing odd about fatigue; we all experience it. There is nothing unusual about headaches, abdominal cramps, achy muscles and joints. Every normal person can understand these symptoms because he or she has experienced them at one time or another. And everyone has had the symptoms of the flu. It is the commonplace nature of the symptoms that suggests a commonplace mechanism causing them. The only thing unusual about the symptoms of CFIDS is that they do not disappear.

A CFIDS-Associated Retrovirus?

If the symptoms of CFIDS result from immune activation, what is the immune system reacting to? The theoretical possibility of a retrovirus as the cause of CFIDS has been discussed for several years, but only recently has any direct evidence linking a retrovirus to this illness been presented. Most hypotheses about this illness have called for a virus of some type to be at least the initiating factor, and from a theoretical point of view, a unique retrovirus makes sense.

The Retrovirus Family

Viruses are divided into different classes based on characteristics that differentiate them. This method of classification occurs with all species. An example is the different types of dogs: They may be divided into different families such as such as collies, German shepherds, poodles, and bulldogs. Each class has certain characteristics that make it unique and separate it from the others. Collies are tall and thin with long hair, bulldogs are short and relatively ugly, and so on.

Among viruses, some are large and have DNA (*d*eoxyribo*n*ucleic *a*cid) for their genetic material, some small and composed of RNA (*r*ibo*n*ucleic *a*cid). Viruses usually carry their own genetic programs with them, and after infecting cells, these programs direct cellular mechanisms to help with multiplication and distribution. Retroviruses are unique in that they merge into the human genetic material, and the human chromosome then directs the proliferation of these agents. The term *retro-* is employed because the programming goes backward into the human DNA.

The structure of a retrovirus is remarkably simple, and the mechanism of action is fiendishly clever. They consist of a single strand of RNA, the genetic program, surrounded by an envelope. The RNA contains the code, called a gene, for several proteins, the most important of which is an enzyme known as reverse transcriptase. This enzyme is not found in any other class of viruses and is responsible for the retro action of retroviruses. It is this enzyme that allows the genetic material of the retrovirus to merge into the human cellular DNA.

After the retrovirus enters the cell, it makes a DNA copy of itself and splices itself into the human chromosome, becoming a provirus. There it looks and acts exactly like the human genetic material. It is no longer really a virus, an outside agent, vulnerable to the immune response. It is now human DNA. It is the perfect spy, forged or counterfeit DNA. But because it is composed of the same materials as the surrounding DNA, it cannot be separated or differentiated from the human chromosome.

This ability to integrate into the host DNA is also responsible for one of the major characteristics of this class of viruses: it can stay hidden and be latent for long periods of time. An infection of a cell with a retrovirus usually does not kill the cell. Indeed, it is to the virus's advantage that the cell stay healthy and function well, since it is conducting business for the retrovirus. Of all the animal and human retroviruses, relatively few are known to cause prominent cell destruction, the most noteworthy being the HIV virus, which causes AIDS. In HIV infection the T4 lymphocyte is destroyed, a cell vital to the immune response, and this usually leads to the death of the AIDS patient.

Another property of retroviruses is that they may alter the host's immune response. There are several reasons for this. While the retrovirus genetic material is hidden in the human chromosome, the body's immune system is not oblivious to the presence of an invader. There are antibodies made to the envelope and other proteins, and the immune system senses the presence of the spy. The ability of the virus to hide in the DNA is analogous to a fly landing on a delicate glass vase. It is not wise to hit the fly with a fly-swatter because the glass will break. Similarly, the host immune response cannot destroy all DNA trying to find the retrovirus because in doing so it will kill itself. Chronic disease with altered immune response and neurologic symptoms are the characteristics of retroviral infection.

Four known retroviruses infect humans: HIV-1 (human immunodeficiency virus 1) is believed to cause AIDS, and HIV-2 is nearly identical to it. HTLV-1 (human T lymphotropic virus 1) causes certain types of leukemias and may cause lymphoma; it has been implicated in multiple sclerosis and other neurologic diseases as well. HTLV-2 (human T lymphotropic virus 2) is also associated with leukemia; little else is known about it.

*C*FIDS *and* AIDS

The similarity between CFIDS and AIDS is an intriguing and controversial topic. Their resemblance is striking, yet both physicians and patients have been very reluctant to notice it. If, in fact, the two illnesses have similarities, it would be worth our time to examine them. The fact that AIDS is caused by a retrovirus could bolster the hypothesis that CFIDS is caused by a retrovirus. Even a hypothetical association could suggest treatment options that may help in research.

It is obvious that major differences exist between AIDS and CFIDS: the lack of severe immune suppression (T4 lymphocyte depletion) and lack of transmission risk factors are the two main factors separating them. No one has seriously suggested that the illnesses are so similar that they may be variations of the same thing. They are clearly separate and distinct illnesses. The most fundamental and striking difference is that CFIDS is not fatal.

Nor are the two illnesses spread by the same route. AIDS is transmitted solely by blood-to-blood contact, meaning that only direct contact with infected blood can transmit the infection from one person to another. This may occur through blood transfusion, sharing hypodermic needles, and sex, particularly homosexual sexual contact. The common thread of blood-to-blood transmission was one of the big clues in the early days of the AIDS epidemic and is not present among patients with CFIDS.

As was discussed in the chapter on the history of CFIDS, there have been many epidemics of CFIDS, and they did not have any common element of blood-to-blood transmission. In fact, most authors studying these epidemics concluded that the spread was through casual contact, such as coughing or sneezing. Furthermore, many children develop CFIDS, children who have never had any exposure to the known means whereby AIDS is spread.

Of the known human retroviruses, none is known to be spread other than through blood-to-blood transmission. Therefore, if we are to postulate that CFIDS is caused by a retrovirus, it must be different from any of the known human retroviruses; it must be one that can be spread by casual contact. If CFIDS is due to retroviral infection, it would have to be a unique retrovirus. Although no such virus is known to infect humans, it is of interest that many of the known animal retroviruses are spread by casual contact. Thus it is not out of the range of possibility that a novel human retrovirus exists.

Despite the important differences between CFIDS and AIDS, let us look at the areas in which the two illnesses are similar.

Flulike Onset

Although it is not generally known, AIDS frequently begins with a flulike illness that may last a few days to several weeks and then resolve. It is felt that this stage represents the initial response of the body to the infection with the HIV virus. In HIV infection, the virus is able to integrate itself into the human DNA and thus disappear from sight, and the flulike symptoms disappear, although the virus is still present. In some patients with HIV infection, the initial flulike onset emerges rapidly into ongoing symptoms, and the patient has AIDS.

In CFIDS the initial flulike infection is well known. Most investigators have stated that up to three-quarters of patients with CFIDS have an initial flulike infection; the remaining have a gradual onset of symptoms, or the symptoms are triggered by some other type of event.

Latency Period

It is likely that the majority of patients with acute flulike onset have their initial contact with the virus at this time, it is also possible that the flulike illness is due to a trigger infection, one that triggers the onset of CFIDS. It is possible that many people who have an initial infection with a hypothetical CFIDS retrovirus have a flulike infection and then become well, only to have the symptoms emerge later with a trigger infection or emerge gradually over a prolonged period of time, much like AIDS develops after the latent HIV infection stage.

Chronic Infection

Most viruses cause an acute infection that resolves after a relatively short illness. This is testimony to the effectiveness of our immune systems in resolving viral infections. But although the symptoms may disappear, not all viruses are completely eradicated from the body; after the initial infection, these viruses cause no symptoms, unless the body's immune system is not functioning properly. Retroviruses, on the other hand, characteristically cause a chronic, ongoing infection that cannot be checked by the normal immune response.

Symptoms

AIDS is one of the illnesses included in the Centers for Disease Control guidelines that must be excluded in patients suspected of having CFIDS. The reason is simple: the symptoms of early AIDS and CFIDS are strikingly similar. Fatigue, fever, sweats, sore throat, lymph node pain, headache, muscle and joint pain, diarrhea, and abdominal discomfort are all shared between the two illnesses. In the later stages of AIDS, profound weight loss, severe secondary infections, and malignancies occur, unlike in CFIDS.

Dementia and Cognitive Problems

Descriptions of the cognitive symptoms present in the two illnesses, particularly in the early stages of AIDS, are virtually identical. Difficulty concentrating, emotional lability, impaired judgment, memory loss, and difficulty with word finding and calculating are all shared symptoms. Other neurologic symptoms, including visual disturbances, weakness, sensory changes, dizziness, abnormal gait, paresthesias, and seizures (only rarely seen in CFIDS), also are similar.

Immune System Involvement

AIDS is well known for the immunodeficiency that is reflected in its name: *a*cquired *i*mmune *d*eficiency *s*yndrome. The most prominent immune deficiency is the loss of the T4 lymphocyte, but there are many other abnormalities, most of which are shared with CFIDS. For example, both illnesses have abnormal immunoglobulin and immunoglobulin subclass levels, decreased cell-mediated immunity, disordered cytokine levels, and circulating immune complexes.

Opportunistic (Reactivated) Viral Infections

Elevated antibody levels to the Epstein-Barr virus and other viruses of the herpes group occur in both CFIDS and AIDS, although they are more severe in the latter. Other secondary infections also are shared, such as yeast infections, but the life-threatening complications of AIDS do not occur in CFIDS. This difference is really one of degree, as the T4 lymphocyte levels do not drop to dangerous levels as they do in AIDS.

A Retroviral Cause for CFIDS?

In 1987 Professor J. C. Murdoch of New Zealand published a letter stating that he believed a retrovirus to be the likely cause of the illness and that he was pursuing further studies (Murdoch 87b). In 1988, Dr. A. Komaroff of Harvard University looked for reverse transcriptase, the enzyme frequently associated with retroviral infections, and was unable to detect it (Komaroff 88). In an oral presentation, Dr. Dharam Ablashi mentioned at the Kansas City CFS Conference in May 1988 that he detected reverse transcriptase in two CFIDS patients, but concluded that it was absent in the majority of patients. Dr. Michael Holmes of New Zealand mentioned his pursuit of reverse transcriptase, detecting it in low concentrations (Cambridge Symposium on Myalgic Encephalomyelitis, 1990). Dr. Daniel Peterson of Incline Village initiated studies with Ampligen, a drug designed originally to treat retroviral infections. It is possible that many other investigators have also entertained the hypothesis of a retrovirus as the cause of this illness.

In a presentation in Kyoto, Japan, Dr. Elaine DeFreitas presented a paper demonstrating retroviral gene sequences found in patients with CFIDS. This paper was a preliminary presentation only and did not prove that a retrovirus was the cause of CFIDS. In fact, it did not even prove that an intact, infective virus was present in these patients. However, the mere presence of the sequences is of interest, and one interpretation of the data could be that a retrovirus was involved in CFIDS. These preliminary data, in combination with the attractive theoretical reasons that CFIDS might be a retroviral disease, have generated excitement and, of course, controversy.

The first study performed was to examine patients with CFIDS to see if they had antibodies to the HTLV-1 and -2 viruses. By the strict criteria used in this study, 41 percent of the thirty patients tested were positive. By itself, 41 percent does not sound very impressive, but considering that this virus is extremely rare and should almost never be found in healthy persons, the finding was of great interest. Now it became important to determine which of the two viruses, HTLV-1 or HTLV-2, was responsible for these positive findings. For this, DeFreitas used a technique called the polymerase chain reaction, or PCR.

The PCR is perhaps the most exciting new technology in medicine. It is possible that within several years it will replace most of the standard means of laboratory diagnosis. There are three main advantages of this technique: (1) it is very sensitive and specific to the organism being tested for; (2) it measures the actual presence of the organism and not just the antibodies formed by the body's immune response; (3) once the procedure is established, it should be relatively inexpensive. Because the genetic codes of both HTLV-1 and HTLV-2 are known, this procedure can probe a patient's blood for their presence. It does this by looking for a specific sequence or arrangement of base pairs, the building blocks of the genetic code.

In her PCR study, DeFreitas chose sequences for the HTLV-1 retrovirus, and all were negative when tested in children and adults with CFIDS. There was no evidence that the HTLV-1 virus was present. Then sequences for the HTLV-2 virus were tried. In the thirty patients, over 75 percent were positive for this specific sequence, implying that HTLV-2 might be present. Moreover, over 30 percent of healthy family members were positive, whereas controls without contact were uniformly negative.

In an attempt to confirm the presence of HTLV-2 virus, another set of sequences was examined from another gene. All patients, contact controls, and noncontact controls were negative for the sequences of this gene. Therefore, the known standard HTLV-2 virus could not be present. One possible explanation for this finding would be that the PCR test was reacting to a new virus, one that was similar to HTLV-2.

This hypothesis is not entirely unreasonable. In the early days of research on AIDS, the first evidence of the presence of a retrovirus was a reaction of AIDS patients' blood to genes of the HTLV-1 virus. It was subsequently discovered that the AIDS virus was unique and that the original reaction to genes of HTLV-1 virus was due to a similarity in this particular region. The similarity between HTLV-1 and HIV in certain genes explained the original positive findings.

The hypothesis that CFIDS is caused by a novel human retrovirus requires an important clarification. As discussed in previous chapters, the symptoms of CFIDS are probably caused by cytokines, the interleukins and interferons. The abnormalities of the cytokines would be caused by the retrovirus. It would then be theoretically possible that many people infected with the CFIDS retrovirus would not have an immunological reaction to it, and thus have no symptoms. People with a genetic tendency to overreact immunologically—that is, to have allergies and/or asthma—are more likely to develop symptoms.

One of the greatest supports to a retroviral theory is that retroviruses are known to be potent stimulators of cytokines, and this is consistent with the theory that cytokines cause the symptoms of CFIDS. Also, there is little or no tissue destruction seen in CFIDS, another characteristic of many retroviral infections. A further, and perhaps the most supportive, trait of retroviruses in general is that they may cause little or no illness. For example, in infections caused by the retrovirus HTLV-1, perhaps the majority of people with this virus have no symptoms at all. It is theoretically possible that the virus does little damage but that symptoms appear only when it stimulates the production of cytokines (Figure 16–1).

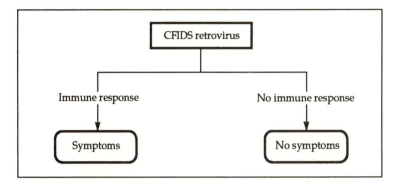

Figure 16–1: If a retrovirus is the underlying cause of CFIDS, then it is possible that the presence of symptoms is determined purely by the immune response generated.

Thus, from a theoretical point of view, I think this theory is the most satisfying of the many options offered over the years. But experimental research is in its infancy and data are unconfirmed. Other laboratories must take up this interesting clue and either confirm it or put it quietly to rest with other unfulfilled dreams. If the results that DeFreitas and her group have published are confirmed, the research will leap into high gear, and it is my hope that the cause and the cure may not be far away.

The Frontier of Twenty-First-Century Medicine

*I*n this book, I have painted a picture of the illness known as chronic fatigue / immune dysfunction syndrome, or CFIDS. Some researchers maintain it is an illness that has been seen for many years yet has eluded scientific research. Others maintain that because of the dramatic nature of the symptoms and prolonged course, this illness could not have escaped the excellent clinicians that practiced medicine prior to sophisticated medical technology. A third group believes that a relatively rare condition, postinfectious fatigue, has always existed, and that we are now seeing an epidemic of an agent or agents that initiate it.

Although this debate cannot be decided without more information, it has become clear that CFIDS is a real and enormous public health problem. No accurate data exist, but it is likely that millions of Americans have CFIDS, some in a mild form, some severe. It is said that the illness is not fatal, but that is not true. The despair that accompanies CFIDS can be so enormous that suicide is a realistic complication, one that can be easily prevented by the understanding and compassion of physicians.

The past five years of research in this country (and thirty years of research in Great Britain) can be viewed from several different perspectives. From the perspective of patients with CFIDS, it has been a nightmare of inattention, apathy, and confusion. They experienced lack of serious approach from their physicians, lack of

231

sympathy from their friends, and lack of compassion from society. They have been the victims of modern medicine, where an inadequate technology has determined that they were neurotic, malingering complainers. They have been the victims of dehumanized physicians who take their orders from machines and laboratory results.

From the perspective of the practicing physician, CFIDS can be a subject of annoyance and frustration. The family physician is isolated, given no help or support by the technology of the specialists. Specialists have been eager to dump CFIDS patients back on their primary physicians, and some family physicians, in an attempt to look more professional, dump their patients by telling them not to return for further appointments. Fortunately, there are thousands of physicians who have continued to try to help patients with CFIDS. They are true physicians who practice the art of medicine without firm answers from technology. Society's respect may have been diverted to machines and technology, but the greater debt is to those physicians who care about their patients.

A third perspective is that of the CFIDS researchers. For me, watching the suffering of patients with CFIDS and enduring the lack of significant response from public health agencies have been frustrating. The slow pace of progress has been agonizing, yet tempered somewhat by the understanding of the caution necessary for accuracy. Medical bureaucracy has an obligation to be careful. But overall, we share complaints with the patients we treat.

There is also a side to this issue that most CFIDS patients don't see. The CFIDS researcher experiences excitement that medical progress is about to make the greatest leap it has ever known. The human body is a huge pyramid in front of us, and in the past many tunnels have been found, unlocking its mysteries. One great tunnel was the discovery of microorganisms, leading to the treatment of infectious illnesses. Another great tunnel was the discovery of genetic structure, leading to the development of molecular biology.

CFIDS is a huge granite block in front of us, appearing impenetrable, standing among thousands of other blocks of the pyramid. But the CFIDS researcher knows that this one block, if it can be moved, will expose a tunnel that will allow huge areas of the pyramid to be explored. It is not only CFIDS that is being understood; the knowledge will affect many other illnesses.

Immune system activation is perhaps the most exciting and productive area in the research on this disease. This area may explain the numerous symptoms of CFIDS. And from the advances made in studying CFIDS, we may be on the edge of understanding such things as the common cold, depression, and tension headaches. Other immune activation diseases, such as sarcoidosis and lupus, may be exposed by the tunnel lying just behind this one block. Psoriasis, rheumatoid arthritis, multiple sclerosis, and endometriosis are just down the tunnel. Cancer may lie at the junction of the CFIDS tunnel and that of molecular biology. The archaeologists working on the other blocks of this pyramid do not believe that a tunnel lies behind the one labeled CFIDS, but CFIDS researchers have heard the subtle echoes that indicate its importance. Despite shouts from the CFIDS researchers, few are willing to listen. The echoes cannot be communicated in scientific terms, yet they are real.

For CFIDS patients the despair they experience makes the full scientific potential of understanding the mechanisms of this illness irrelevant. They are not concerned about rheumatoid arthritis or multiple sclerosis. Their suffering is the neglected physical discomfort of the illness and their despair is over their neglect by physicians and society. For CFIDS researchers, the suffering we witness in our patients is motivation enough. Moving the block labeled CFIDS has always been, and remains, the goal.

At the time of this writing, it has been nearly eight years since the original descriptions of CFIDS in this country appeared. Yet the official response has been negligible, microscopic amounts of funding allocated for research. The denial of public health officials has taken the form of trivializing CFIDS and ridiculing those suffering from it. Public health officials have pretended ignorance to excuse inaction while knowledge of the illness exists. The official response to CFIDS has been to put patients and researchers on the defensive. It is not just a question of money. Mere scientific encouragement would have helped. But those times have passed, and that opportunity was missed.

With the knowledge presently gained about CFIDS, public health agencies no longer need to begin from scratch. They can no longer maintain the illusion of ignorance, because medical journals are filling with important data. Trivialization of the illness will no longer be tolerated by patients or their physicians. What is now necessary is cooperation and the spending of the research money required for the next phase of research. And it is clear that changes in the old attitudes have begun.

As a CFIDS researcher, I would like to see billions of dollars poured into research. The economic losses of productive Americans being unable to work because of CFIDS are staggering. The despair and suffering they experience cannot be measured. Because of the devastation of the illness, part of me feels that every American should be taxed five, ten, or fifteen dollars a year for CFIDS research. But we also have to be realistic.

From the public health standpoint, the needs are simple. Take the clues already present concerning CFIDS and determine the cause. Then we will know our enemy. We will be able to develop markers to diagnose the illness easily, treatment strategies, means of prevention, and perhaps a vaccine. CFIDS is not an insoluble problem. The frustration that many researchers feel is that these answers are so close. We know the basic mechanisms, but a new and deeper level of research is needed to work out the details. And this is not an untreatable condition. I have great optimism that with a little more knowledge, the immune abnormalities that cause the symptoms of CFIDS can be safely bypassed. I also believe that the cause or causes of these immune system changes can be accurately defined and treated. But before this will happen, perceptions must change.

As a society, we are comfortable in the belief that we are insulated. Our emotional defenses are active in creating and protecting this insulation. With the advent of technology and the rapid and accurate spread of information, we have become aware of the enormous crises that exist for us as a society. We know that our waters are polluted, that atomic weapons exist with the potential to anni-hilate all living creatures, that toxic chemicals are poured into the air, that drugs are eroding the fabric of our society. We know of AIDS and its devastation of central Africa, threatening to do the same to North America. We know our enemies and yet do nothing. The greater the horror we see threatening us, the more we wish to pretend it does not exist. We bind ourselves in an emotional insulation that gives strength to our enemies. We have stopped struggling to defend ourselves, and we are losing the qualities that make us human.

We have developed the habit of sitting within our houses, watching television, pretending not to notice the hurricane blow-ing at our door. A part of each of us is aware that we must fight, but a competing part overwhelms us with apathy. We are afraid of the hurricane and try to escape to the solace of our fantasy. We have the ability to fight our enemies, but we are unwilling to. We are like Nero, fiddling while Rome burns. We don't want to put aside our useless denials and face the challenges before us. And the reason is simple: we are afraid that if we struggle against our enemies, our present comfort will be compromised. We wish to preserve every moment of our present comfort, even if it en-sures our destruction as a society.

While patients suffering the despair of CFIDS may disagree, I do not feel that CFIDS is our greatest enemy. Our enemy is the apathy that has allowed CFIDS to go unrecognized, the same apathy that has allowed our society to fall to the present dangerous level. My strongest wish is that we open our eyes to what sur-rounds us, examine our enemies, and at least begin to fight against them. We should put aside our fantasies but not our hopes. We should accept the challenge of trying to survive, even if this re-quires setting aside our transient comforts.

In regard to CFIDS, the need is simple. It is not billions of dollars for medical research, for those billions have more urgent needs; CFIDS is a horrible illness, but it is not as dangerous as AIDS or cancer. And no one is asking the family physician to cure the patient with CFIDS—it cannot be done with the present technology. Instead, I ask that physicians drop their arrogance and denial and offer help to their patients. Abandon the silly argument of whether CFIDS is a real disease, talk to those suffering with it, and treat them with the same respect that is given to patients with other illnesses. Every practicing physician probably has at least one CFIDS patient in his or her practice. For the average patient with CFIDS who is struggling to remain a productive member of society, respect alone will alleviate half of the suffering.

And to those who suffer from CFIDS, look beyond the limitations of today's medicine. Progress continues toward the day when CFIDS can join the legions of diseases that modern medicine has conquered.

CFIDS Questionnaire

Please mark an "x" next to the number that most closely represents the amount of pain or difficulty you have for each of the symptoms listed below. It should be representative of a typical day over the past month.

From 0 to 10, how much fatigue, tiredness, or exhaustion do you experience?

	None			Mild		Moderate		Severe		Very Severe
0	1	2	3	4	5	6	7	8	9	10

How much of a problem is sore throat?

	None			Mild		Moderate		Severe		Very Severe
0	1	2	3	4	5	6	7	8	9	10

How severe are headaches?

	None			Mild		Moderate		Severe		Very Severe
0	1	2	3	4	5	6	7	8	9	10

How much of a problem is aching of the eyes, blurry vision, or light sensitivity?

	None			Mild		Moderate		Severe		Very Severe
0	1	2	3	4	5	6	7	8	9	10

How much of a problem is abdominal pain, bloating, or gas?

	None			Mild		Moderate		Severe		Very Severe
0	1	2	3	4	5	6	7	8	9	10

How much of a problem is pain in your lymph nodes?

	None			Mild		Moderate		Severe		Very Severe
0	1	2	3	4	5	6	7	8	9	10

How much of a problem is depression, mood changes, or panic attacks?

	None			Mild		Moderate		Severe		Very Severe
0	1	2	3	4	5	6	7	8	9	10

How much of a problem is pain or aching in your muscles?

	None			Mild		Moderate		Severe		Very Severe
0	1	2	3	4	5	6	7	8	9	10

How much of a problem is memory loss or difficulty concentrating?

	None			Mild		Moderate		Severe		Very Severe
0	1	2	3	4	5	6	7	8	9	10

How much of a problem is poor sleep, insomnia, or waking unrefreshed?

	None			Mild		Moderate		Severe		Very Severe
0	1	2	3	4	5	6	7	8	9	10

How much concern is numbness tingling, dizziness, or balance problems?

	None			Mild		Moderate		Severe		Very Severe
0	1	2	3	4	5	6	7	8	9	10

How much of a problem is pain in your joints?

	None			Mild		Moderate		Severe		Very Severe
0	1	2	3	4	5	6	7	8	9	10

References

Abbey S, Garfinkel PE. Neurasthenia and chronic fatigue syndrome: the role of culture in making of a diagnosis. Am J Psychiatry 1991a; 148(12):1638–46.

Abbey SE, Garfinkel PE. Chronic fatigue syndrome and the psychiatrist. Can J Psychiat 1990; 35(7):625–33.

Abbey SE, Garfinkel PE. Chronic fatigue syndrome and depression: cause, effect, or covariate. Rev Inf Dis 1991b; 13(Suppl 1):S73–83.

Abo W, Takada K, Kamada M, Imamura M, Motoya T, Iwanga M, Aya T, Yano S, Nakao T, Osato T. Evolution of infectious mononucleosis into Epstein-Barr virus carrying monoclonal malignant lymphoma. Lancet 1982; 1:1272–4.

Acheson ED. The clinical syndrome variously called benign myalgic encephalo-myelitis, Iceland disease, and epidemic neuromyasthenia. Am J Med 1959; 26:569–95.

Adolphe AB. Chronic fatigue syndrome: possible effective treatment with nife-dipine. Am J Med 1988; 85:892.

Alexander EL, Kumar AJ, Kozachuk WE. Chronic fatigue syndrome controversy [letter]. Ann Intern Med 1992; 117(4):343–4.

Alfieri C, Ghibu F, Joncas JH. Lytic, nontransforming Epstein-Barr virus (EBV) from a patient with chronic active EBV infection. Can Med Assoc J 1984; 131:1249–52.

Ali M. Ascorbic acid reverses abnormal erythrocyte morphology in chronic fatigue syndrome. Am J Clin Path 1991; 94.

Allen DA. Is RA27/3 Rubella Immunization a cause of chronic fatigue? Med Hypoth 1988; 27:217–20.

Altay HT, Toner BB, Brooker H, Abbey SE, Salit IE, Garfinkel PE. The neuro-psychological dimensions of post-infectious neuromyasthenia (chronic fatigue syndrome): a preliminary report. Int'l J Psychiatry in Med 1990; 20(2):141–9.

Andre, M, Matz B. HHV-6 and chronic fatigue syndrome. [letter] Lancet 17 Dec 1988; 1426.

Aoki T, Usuda Y, Miyakoshi H, Tamura K, Herberman RB. Low natural killer syndrome: clinical and immunologic features. Nat Immun Cell Growth Regul 1987; 6:116–28.

Archard LC, Bowles NE, Behan PO, Bell EJ, Doyle D. Postviral fatigue syndrome: persistence of enterovirus RNA in muscle and elevated creatine kinase. J Roy Soc Meds 1988; 81:326–9.

239

Archer L. The post-infectious chronic fatigue syndrome: virologic studies. *In* Epstein-Barr virus and human disease, eds Ablashi DV et al, Humana Press, 1989; 427-9.

Archer MI. The post viral fatigue syndrome: a review. J Roy Col Gen Pract 1987; 37:212-4.

Armon C, Kurland LT. Chronic fatigue syndrome: issues in the diagnosis and estimation of incidence. Rev Inf Dis 1991; 13 (Suppl 1):S68-72.

Arnason BGW. Nervous system-immune system communication. Rev Inf Dis 1991; 13(Suppl 1):S112-3.

Arnold D, Bore P, Radda G, Styles P, Taylor D. Excessive intracellular acidosis of skeletal muscle on exercise in a patient with post viral exhaustion/fatigue syndrome. Lancet 1985; i:1367-9.

Bakheit AMO, Behan PO, Dinan TG, Gray CE, O'Keane V. Possible upregulation of hypothalamic 5-hydroxytryptamine receptors in patients with postviral fatigue syndrome. BMJ 1992; 304:1010-2.

Ballow M, Seeley J, Purtilo JT, Onge BS, Sakamoto K, Rickles FR. Familial chronic mononucleosis. Ann Intern Med 1982; 97:821-5.

Barnes DM. Mystery disease at Lake Tahoe challenges virologists and clinicians. Science 1986; 234:541-2.

Barofsky I, Legro MW. Definition and measurement of fatigue. Rev Inf Dis 1991; 13(Suppl 1):S94-7.

Bass C. Fatigue states [editorial]. Br J Hosp Med Apr 1989; 41(4):315.

Bates T, Grunwaldt E. Myofascial pain in childhood. J Pediatr 1958; 53:198-209.

Becker JT. Methodologic considerations in assessment of cognitive function in chronic fatigue syndrome. Rev Inf Dis 1991; 13(Suppl 1):S112-3.

Behan PO. Post viral neurological syndromes. BMJ 1983; 287:2871.

Behan PO, Behan WMH. Epidemic myalgic encephalitis. *In* Clinical neouroepidemiology, ed Clifford F, Pitmans, 1980; 374-83.

Behan PO, Behan WMH. Postviral fatigue syndrome. CRC (Critical Reviews in Neurobiology) 1988a; 4:2157-178.

Behan PO, Behan WMH. Myalgic encephalomyelitis. Nightingale Research Foundation, Ottawa, Canada, 1988b.

Behan PO, Behan WMH. Essential fatty acids in the treatment of postviral fatigue syndrome. Omega-6 essential fatty acids: pathophysiology and roles in clinical medicine, Alan R. Liss, Inc, 1990; 275-82.

Behan PO, Behan WMH, Bell EJ. The post-viral fatigue syndrome—an analysis of findings in 50 cases. J Infect 1985; 10:211-22.

Behan PO, Goldberg DP, Mowbray JF, eds. Postviral fatigue syndrome. Br Med Bull 1991; 47:4.

Behan WMH. Muscles, mitochondria and myalgia. J Path 1992; 166:213–4.

Behan WMH, More IAR, Behan PO. Mitochondrial abnormalities in the postviral fatigue syndrome. Acta Neuropathologica 1991; 83:61–5.

Bell DS. Children with ME/CFIDS: Overview and review of the literature. *In* The clinical and scientific basis of myalgic encephalomyelitis chronic fatigue syndrome, ed Hyde BM, Nightingale Research Foundation, Ottawa, Canada, 1992a; 209–18.

Bell DS. Chronic fatigue syndrome: recent advances in diagnosis and treatment. Postgrad Med 1992b; 91(6):245–52.

Bell DS. The chronic fatigue syndrome [letter]. Am J Psychiatry 1992c; 149:1753.

Bell DS, Bell KM. Chronic fatigue syndrome: diagnostic criteria [letter]. Ann Intern Med 1988; 109(2):167.

Bell DS, Bell KM. The post-infectious chronic fatigue syndrome: diagnosis in childhood. *In* Epstein-Barr virus and human disease, eds Ablashi DV et al, Humana Press, 1989; 412–7.

Bell EJ, McCartney RA, Riding MH. Coxsackie B viruses and myalgic encephalomyelitis. J Roy Soc Med 1988; 81:329.

Bell KM, Cookfair D, Reese P, Bell D, Cooper L. Risk factors with chronic fatigue syndrome in children [abstract]. Am J Epidemiol 1988; 128:899.

Bell KM, Cookfair D, Bell DS, Reese P, Cooper L. Risk factors associated with chronic fatigue syndrome in a cluster of pediatric cases. Rev Inf Dis 1991; 13(Suppl 1): S32–8.

Bender CE. Recurrent mononucleosis. JAMA 1962; 182:954–6.

Bennett RB. Etiology of the fibromyalgia syndrome: a contemporary hypothesis. IM 1990; 11(5):46–61.

Bennett RM. Confounding features of the fibromyalgia syndrome: a current perspective of the differential diagnosis. J Rheumatol Suppl 1988; 19:58–61.

Bennett RM, Leibovitch ER. Chronic fatigue syndrome: new insights in diagnosis and office management. Modern Medicine 1990; 58:50–62.

Bode L, Komaroff AL, Ludwig H. No serologic evidence of Borna disease virus in patients with chronic fatigue syndrome. CID 1992; 15(6):1049.

Boriysiewicz LK, Hayworth SJ, Cohen J, Mundin J, Rickinson A, Sissons JGP. Epstein-Barr specific immune defects in patients with persistent symptoms following infectious mononucleosis. Quart J Med 1986; 58:111–21.

Bowman SJ, Brostoff J, Newman S, Mowbray JF. Postviral syndromes—how can a diagnosis be made? A study of patients undergoing a monospot test. J R Soc Med 1989; 82(12):712–6.

Bradley CA. Psychiatric diagnoses and chronic fatigue syndrome [letter]. J Clin Psychiat 1990; 51(2):86.

Brunell PA. The chronic fatigue syndrome [editorial]. Inf Dis in Children 1989; 2:6.

Buchwald D. The post-infectious chronic fatigue syndrome: laboratory abnormalities. *In* Epstein-Barr virus and human disease, eds Ablashi DV et al, Humana Press, 1989; 419–27.

Buchwald D, Cheney PR, Peterson DL, Henry B, Wormsley SB, Geiger A, Ablashi DV, Salahuddin SZ, Saxinger C, Biddle R, Kikinis R, Jolesz FA, Folks T, Balachandran N, Peter JB, Gallo RC, Komaroff AL. A chronic illness characterized by fatigue, neurologic and immunologic disorders, and active human herpes virus type 6 infection. Ann Intern Med 1992; 116:103–13.

Buchwald D, Freedman AS, Ablashi DV, Sullivan JL, Caligiuri M, Weinberg DS, et al. A chronic "postinfectious" fatigue syndrome associated with benign lymphoproliferation, B-cell proliferation, and active replication of human herpes virus-6. J Clin Immunol 1990; 10:335–44.

Buchwald D, Gantz NM, Katon WJ, Manu P (Gregory T, ed). Tips on chronic fatigue syndrome. Patient Care 1991; 25:45–58.

Buchwald D, Goldenberg DL, Sullivan JL, Komaroff AL. The "chronic active Epstein-Barr virus infection" syndrome and primary fibromyalgia. Arth & Rheum 1987.

Buchwald D, Komaroff AL. Review of laboratory findings for patients with chronic fatigue syndrome. Rev Inf Dis 1991; 13(Suppl 1):S12–8.

Buchwald D, Sullivan JL, Komaroff AL. Frequency of "chronic active Epstein-Barr virus infection" in a general medical practice. JAMA 1987; 257:2303–7.

Buchwald D, Wener MH, Komaroff AL. Antineuronal antibody levels in chronic fatigue syndrome patients with neurologic abnormalities. Arth & Rheum 1991; 34:1485–6.

Butler S, Calder T, Ron M, et al. Cognitive behavior therapy in chronic fatigue syndrome. J Neurol Neurosurg Psychiatry 1991; 54:153–8.

Byrne E. Idiopathic chronic fatigue and myalgia syndrome (myalgic encephalomyelitis): some thoughts on nomenclature and etiology. Med J Aust 1988; 148:80–82.

Byrne E, Trounce I. Chronic fatigue and myalgia syndrome: mitochondrial and glycolytic studies in skeletal muscle. J Neurol Neurosurg Psychiat 1987; 50:743–6.

Cabral DA, Petty RE, Fung M, Malleson PN. Persistent antinuclear antibodies in children without identifiable inflammatory rheumatic or autoimmune disease. Pediatrics 1992; 89:441–4.

Calabrese LH, Danao T, Camara E, Wilke W. Chronic fatigue syndrome. American Family Physician 1992; 45:1205–13.

Calabrese LH, Danao T, Camara EG, Wilke WS. Chronic fatigue and immune dysfunction. Cleveland Clinic J of Med 1992; 59(2):123–4.

Calabro JJ. Fibromyalgia (fibrositis) in children. Am J Med 1986; 81(Suppl 3A):57–9.

Calder BD, Warnock PJ. Chronic fatigue syndrome [letter]. J Roy Soc Med 1991; 83(10):675–6.

Calder BD, Warnock PJ, McCartney RA, Bell EJ. Coxsackie B viruses and the postviral fatigue syndrome: a prospective study in general practice. J R Coll Gen Pract 1987; 37:11–4.

Caligiuri M, Murray C, Buchwald D, Levine H, Cheney P, Peterson D, et al. Phenotypic and functional deficiency of natural killer cells in patients with chronic fatigue syndrome. J Immunol 1987; 139:3306–13.

Camus F, Henzel D, Janowski M, Raguin G, Leport C, Vilde JL. Unexplained fever and chronic fatigue: abnormal circadian temperature pattern. European J of Med 1992; 1:30–36.

Caro XJ. New concepts in primary fibrositis syndrome. Compr Ther May 1989; 15(5):14–22.

Carroll N, Gibson H, Coakley J, Edwards RHT. Cycle ergometry in patients with chronic fatigue syndromes. European Journal of Clinical Investigation 1990; 20 (A29) Abs 148.

Caruso I, Sarzi Puttini P, Cazzola M, Azzolini V. Double blind study of 5-hydroxytryptophan versus placebo in the treatment of primary fibromyalgia syndrome. J Int Med Res 1990; 18(3):201–9.

Cassel W, Archer-Duste H. The new epidemic: chronic fatigue syndrome. Pennsylvania Nurse 1991; 46 (2):8–9.

Cathebras P, Charmion S, Gonthier R, Rousset H, Robbins J. Chronic fatigue, viruses, and depression. Lancet 1991; 337:564–5.

Chang RS. Chronic fatigue syndrome [letter]. JAMA 1991; 265:357.

Chang RS, Maddock R. Recurrence of infectious mononucleosis. Lancet 1978, 2:231–4.

Chao CC, DeLahunt M, Hu S, Close K, Peterson PK. Immunologically mediated fatigue—a murine model. Clinical Immunology and Immunopathology 1992; 64(2):161–6.

Chao CC, Gallagher M, Phair J, Peterson PK. Serum neopterin and interleukin-6 in chronic fatigue syndrome [letter]. JID 1990; 162(6):1412–3.

Cheney PR, Dorman SE, Bell DS. Interleukin-2 and the chronic fatigue syndrome [letter]. Ann Intern Med 1989; 110:321.

Cheverton DPD. Tetracyclines in myalgic encephalomyelitis. South African Medical Journal 1992; 82:369–70.

Cho WK, Stollerman GH. Chronic fatigue syndrome. Hospital Practice 1992; 27(9):119–35.

Chronic Fatigue Syndrome. 1992 Ciba Foundation Symposium. Chichester: Wiley & Sons, London, 1993.

Cicuttini F, Littlejohn GO. Female adolescent rheumatological presentations: the importance of chronic pain syndromes. Aust Paediatr J 1989; 25:21-4.

Clague JE, Edwards RHT, Jackson MJ. Intravenous magnesium loading in chronic fatigue syndrome. Lancet 1992; 340:124-5.

Cluff LE. Medical aspects of delayed convalescence. Rev Inf Dis 1991; 13(Suppl 1):S138-40.

Cookfair DL, Shirley M, Bell DS, Shock B, Rosenthal A. Patient/family education using a support group framework (abstract). J Ca Ed 1988; 4:286.

Corey L, Sixby J. Chronic fatigue syndrome [letter]. JAMA 1991; 265:358.

Costa DC, Brostoff J, Douli V, Ell PJ. Postviral fatigue syndrome. Brit Med J 1992; 304:1567.

Cotton P. Treatment proposed for chronic fatigue syndrome; research continues to compile data on disorder. JAMA 1991; 266:2667.

Cox IM, Campbell MJ, Dowson D. Red blood cell magnesium and chronic fatigue syndrome. Lancet 1991a; 337:757-60.

Cox IM, Campbell MJ, Dowson D. Magnesium and chronic fatigue syndrome [letter]. Lancet 1991b; 337:1295.

Cunha BA. Crimson crescents—a possible association with the chronic fatigue syndrome [letter]. Ann Intern Med 1992; 116:347.

Cunningham L, Bowles NE, Lane RJ, Dubowitz V, Archard LC. Persistence of enteroviral RNA in chronic fatigue syndrome is associated with abnormal production of equal amounts of positive and negative strands of enteroviral RNA. J Gen Virol 1990; 71(6):1399-402.

Cuozzo J. Chronic fatigue [letter]. JAMA 1989; 261:697.

DaCosta Brostoff J, Douli V, Ell PJ. Brain stem hypoperfusion in patients with myalgic encephalomyelitis—chronic fatigue syndrome. European Journal of Nuclear Medicine 1992; 19(8):733.

Dale JK, DiBisceglie AM, Hoofnagle JH, Straus SE. Chronic fatigue syndrome: lack of association with hepatitis C virus infection. Journal of Med Virol 1991; 34:119-21.

Dale JK, Straus SE, Ablashi D, Salahuddin ZS, Gallo RC, Nishibe Y, Inoue YK. The Inoue-Melnik virus, human herpes virus type 6 and the chronic fatigue syndrome [letter]. Ann Intern Med 1989; 110:92-3.

Dalgleish AG. Immunological abnormalities in the chronic fatigue syndrome [letter]. Med J Aust 1990; 152:50.

Daugherty SA, Henry BE, Peterson DL, Swarts RL, Bastien S, Thomas RS. Chronic fatigue syndrome in northern Nevada. Rev Inf Dis 1991; 13(Suppl 1):S39-44.

David AS, Wessely S, Pelosi AJ. Postviral fatigue syndrome: time for a new approach. BMJ 1988; 296:696-9.

Dawson J. Royal Free disease: perplexity continues. Br Med J 1987; 294:327-8.

DeFreitas E, Hilliard B, Cheney P, Bell D, Kiggundu E, Sankey D, Wroblewska Z, Koprowski H. Evidence of retrovirus in patients with chronic fatigue immune dysfunction syndrome [abstract]. Proceedings of the XIth International Congress of Neuropathology, Kyoto, Japan, Sept 1990.

DeFreitas E, Hilliard B, Cheney P, Bell D, Kiggundu E, Sankey D, Wroblewska Z, Palladino M, Woodward JP, Koprowski H. Retroviral sequences related to human T-lymphotropic virus type II in patients with chronic fatigue immune dysfunction syndrome. Proc Natl Acad Sci 1991; 88:2922-26.

DeFreitas E, Koprowski H. Statements regarding chronic fatigue immune dysfunction syndrome to the US House of Representatives committee on energy and commerce, subcommittee on health and the environment. 16 Apr 1991.

Demitrack MA, Dale JK, Straus SE, Laue L, Listwak SJ, Kruesi MJP, Chrousos GP, Gold PW. Evidence for impaired activation of the hypothalamic-pituitary-adrenal axis in patients with chronic fatigue syndrome. J Clin Endocrinol Metab 1991; 73:1224-34.

Demitrack MA, Greden JF. Chronic fatigue syndrome: the need for an integrative approach. Bio Psychiat 1991; 30:747-52.

Dillon MJ. Epidemic neuromyasthenia at the Hospital for sick children, Great Ormond Street. London. Postgrad Med J 1978; 54:757-64, 814-18.

Doepel LK. Lifetime history of psychiatric illness in people with chronic fatigue syndrome. Update—National Institute of Allergy and Infectious Diseases, 15 Feb 1989.

Donald P. Chronic Epstein-Barr virus syndrome. The Bulletin of the Amer Acad of Otolaryngology and Neck Surgery (AAO-HNS Bulletin) 1988; 7:11-2.

Donald PJ. Chronic mononucleosis in adults. West J Med Feb 1987; 146:249.

Dooley DP. Commercial laboratory testing for chronic fatigue syndrome. JAMA 1992; 268:873-4.

Douglas W. Immunological abnormalities in the chronic fatigue syndrome [letter]. Med J Aust 1990; 152:50.

Douli V, Brostoff J, Costa CD, Kouris K, Ell PJ. rCBF/SPET in patients with myalgic encephalomyelitis. Nuclear Medicine Communications [Abstract of 20th ann meeting of British Nuclear Medicine Society] 1992; 13:4.

Downey DC. Fatigue syndromes: new thoughts and reinterpretation of previous data. Medical Hypothesis 1992; 39(2):185-90.

Dowsett EG, Ramsay AM, McCartney RA, Bell EJ. Myalgic encephalomyelitis—a persistent viral infection? Postgrad Med J 1990; 66:526-30.

DuBois RE. Gamma globulin therapy for chronic mononucleosis syndrome. AIDS Research 1986; 1(suppl):S191-5.

246   *The Doctor's Guide to Chronic Fatigue Syndrome*

Dubois RE. The post-infectious chronic fatigue syndrome: discussion. *In* Epstein-Barr virus and human disease, eds Ablashi DV et al, Humana Press, 1989; 417-9.

DuBois RE, Seeley JK, Brus I, Sakamoto K, Ballow M, Harada S, Bechtold TA, Pearson G, Purtilo DT. Chronic mononucleosis syndrome. South Med J 1984; 77:1376-82.

Durlach J. Chronic fatigue syndrome and chronic primary magnesium deficiency (CFS and CPMD). Magnesium Research 1992; 5(1):68.

Dwyer B. Chronic fatigue: a new immunosuppressive virus? The Psychiatric Times July 1987; Vol IV; 7:1-4.

Dwyer JM, Lloyd A, Wakefield D, Boughton C. Gamma Globulin for chronic fatigue syndrome? A treatment and a clue. Patient Management Nov 1988; 157-60.

Edwards BL, Bonagura VR, Valacer DJ, Ilowite NT. Mucha-Habermann's disease and arthritis: possible association with reactivated Epstein-Barr virus infection. J Reumatol 1989 Mar; 16(3):387-9.

Edwards L, Ray CG, Meltzer P, Litwin CM, Sobonya RE, Chipowsky S. Wasting disease associated with Epstein-Barr virus infection. Pediatr Infect Dis J 1988; 7:719-24.

Eichner ER. Chronic fatigue syndrome: drug and non-drug treatment. Drug Therapy Aug 1990; 29-38.

Elnicki DM, Shockcor WT, Brick JA, Benyon D. Evaluating the complaint of fatigue in primary care: diagnoses and outcomes. Am J Med 1992; 93:303-6.

English T. A piece of my mind: skeptical of skeptics. JAMA 1991; 265:964.

Evans AS. Chronic fatigue syndrome: thoughts on pathogenesis. Rev Inf Dis 1991; 13(Suppl 1):S56-9.

Fark AR. Infectious mononucleosis, Epstein-Barr virus, and chronic fatigue syndrome: a prospective case series. J Fam Pract 1991; 32(2):202, 205-6, 209.

Fegan KG, Behan PO, Bell EJ. Myalgic encephalomyelitis—report of an epidemic. J Roy Col Gen Pract 1983; 33:335-7.

Fleisher G, Bolognese R. Persistent Epstein-Barr virus infection and pregnancy. J Inf Dis 1983; 147:982-6.

Fletcher MA, Klimas N. Chronic fatigue syndrome [letter]. JAMA 1991; 265:357.

Flugel RM, Mahnke C, Geiger A, Komaroff AL. Absence of antibody to human spumaretrovirus in patients with chronic fatigue syndrome. CID 1992; 14:623-4.

Franco E, Kawa-ha K, Doi S, Yumura K, Murata M, Ishihara S, Tawa A, Yabuuchi H. Remarkable depression of CD4+2H4+ T cells in severe chronic active Epstein-Barr virus infection. Scand J Immunol 1987 26:769-73.

Fuchs D, Weiss G, Wachter H. Pathogenesis of chronic fatigue syndrome. J Clin Psychiat 1992; 53:296.

Furman JMR. Testing of vestibular function: an adjunct in the assessment of chronic fatigue syndrome. Rev Inf Dis 1991; 13(Suppl 1):S109–11.

Gantz NM. Magnesium and chronic fatigue. Lancet 1991; 338:66.

Gantz NM. An update of chronic fatigue syndrome. Contemporary Internal Medicine April 1992; 53–67.

Gantz NM, Holmes GP. Treatment of patients with chronic fatigue syndrome. Drugs 1989; 38(6):855–62.

Gerow G, Poierier MB, Alt R. Chronic fatigue syndrome. Journal of Manipulative and Physiological Therapeutics. 1992; 15(8):529–35.

Gibson H, Carroll N, Coakley J, Edwards RHT. Recovery from maximal exercises in chronic fatigue states. European Journal of Clinical Investigation 1990; 20, A29, Abs 147.

Gill CR. Myalgic encephalitis [letter]. Practitioner 1990; 61(7):390–6.

Gin W, Christiansen FT, Peter JB. Immune function and the chronic fatigue syndrome. Med J Aust 1989; 151(3):117–8.

Gold D, Bowden R, Sixbey J, Riggs R, Katon WJ, Ashley R, Obrigewitch RM, Corey L. Chronic fatigue—a prospective clinical and virologic study. JAMA 1990; 264(1):48–53.

Goldenberg DL. Fibromyalgia and other chronic fatigue syndromes: is there evidence for chronic viral disease? Sem Arth Rheum 1988; 18:2:111–20.

Goldenberg DL. Fibromyalgia and its relation to chronic fatigue syndrome, viral illness, and immune abnormalities. J Reumatol Suppl 1989; 19:91–3.

Goldenberg DL. Fibromyalgia, chronic fatigue syndrome and myofascial pain syndrome. Cur Opin Rheum 1991; 3:247–58.

Goldenberg DL, Simms RW, Geiger A, Komaroff AL. High frequency of fibromyalgia in patients with chronic fatigue seen in a primary care practice. Arth & Rheum 1990; 33(3):381–7.

Goldstein J. Chronic fatigue syndrome. The Female Patient 1991; 16:35–50.

Goldstein K, Lai PK, Lightfoot EM, et al. Relationship of in vitro immune responses to Epstein-Barr herpes virus and severity of infectious mononucleosis. Infect Immun 1980; 29:945–52.

Goodnick PJ. Bupropion in chronic fatigue syndrome [letter]. An J Psychiat 1990; 147(8):1091.

Goodnick PJ, Sandoval R. Psychotropic treatment of chronic fatigue syndrome and related disorders. J Clin Psychiat 1993; 54:13–20.

Gordon, N. Myalgic encephalomyelitis. Dev Med & Child Neurol 1988; 30:673–82.

Gow JW, Behan WMH, Clements GB, Woodall C, Riding M, Behan PO. Enteroviral RNA sequences detected by polymerase chain reaction in muscle of patients with postviral fatigue syndrome. BMJ 1991; 302:692–96.

Gracious B, Wisner KL. Nortriptyline in chronic fatigue syndrome: a double-blind, placebo-controlled single case study. Biol Psychiat 1991; 30:405–8.

Grafman J, Johnson R, Scheffers M. Cognitive and mood-state changes in patients with chronic fatigue syndrome. Rev Inf Dis 1991; 13(Suppl 1):S45–52.

Grau JM, Casademont J, Pedrol E, Fernandez-Sola J, Cardellach F, Barros N, Urbano-Marquez A. Chronic fatigue syndrome: studies on skeletal muscle. Clin Neuropath 1992; 11(6):329–32.

Graves S. Recurrent Infectious mononucleosis. J Ky Med Assoc 1970; 1:790–2.

Greenberg DB. Neurasthenia in the 1980s. Psychosomatics 1990; 31(2):129–37.

Griffin DE. Immunologic abnormalities accompanying acute and chronic viral infections. Rev Inf Dis 1991; 13(Suppl 1):S129–33.

Grist NR. Myalgic encephalomyelitis: postviral fatigue syndrome and the heart [letter]. BMJ 1989; 299 (6709):1219.

Grufferman S. Issues and problems in the conduct of epidemiologic research on chronic fatigue syndrome. Rev Inf Dis 1991; 13(Suppl 1):S60–7.

Grufferman S, Eby NL, Huang M, Whiteside T, Sumaya CV, Saxinger WC, Herberman RB. Epidemiologic investigation of an outbreak of chronic fatigue-immune dysfunction syndrome in a defined population [abstract]. Am J Epidemiol 1988; 128:898.

Gunn WJ, Komaroff AL, Bell DS, Connell DB, Levine SM, Cheney PR. Inability of retroviral tests to identify persons with chronic fatigue syndrome, 1992. MMWR 19 March 1993; 42:183–90.

Gupta S, Vayuvegula B. Comprehensive immunological analysis in chronic fatigue syndrome. Scand J Immunol 1991; 33:319–27.

Gurwitt A, Barrett S, Brown S, Butaney ECA, Gorman B, Kilgore JL, O'Grady E, Potaznick W, Saltzstein B, Sanford A, Webster W, Zimmer V. Chronic fatigue syndrome: a primer for physicians and allied health professionals, Massachusetts CFIDS Society, Waltham, Mass., 1992.

Halpin D, Wessely S. VP-1 antigen in chronic post-viral fatigue syndrome [letter]. Lancet 1989; 1(8645):1028–9.

Hamblin JT, Hussain J, Akbar AN, et al. Immunological reason for chronic ill health after infectious mononucleosis. Br Med J Clin Res 1983; 287:85–8.

Harris F, Taitz LS. Damaging diagnosis of myalgic encephalomyelitis in children [letter]. BMJ 1989; 299(6702):790.

Hartwell L. Post viral fatigue syndrome: a canker in my brain [letter]. Lancet 1987; i:910.

Hellinger WC, Smith TF, Van Scoy RE, Spitzer PG, Forgacs P, Edson RS. Chronic fatigue syndrome and the diagnostic utility of antibody to Epstein-Barr virus early antigen. JAMA 1988; 260:971–3.

Hench PK. Evaluation and differential diagnosis of fibromyalgia. Approach to diagnosis and management. Rheum Clin NA 1989; 15:19–29.

Henderson DA, Shelokov A. Epidemic neuromyasthenia—clinical syndrome. N Eng J Med 1959; 260:757–64.

Herberman RB. Sources of confounding in immunologic data. Rev Inf Dis 1991; 13(Suppl 1):S84–6.

Hermann WJ. The Epstein-Barr virus and chronic fatigue syndrome [letter]. 1989; 261:1277–8.

Hickie I, Lloyd A, Wakefield D, Parker G. The psychiatric status of patients with chronic fatigue syndrome. Br J Psychiat 1990; 156:534–40.

Hickie I, Lloyd A, Wakefield D. Immunological and psychological dysfunction in patients receiving immunotherapy for chronic fatigue syndrome. Australian and New Zealand Journal of Psychiatry 1992; 26(2):249–56.

Hilgers A, Frank J. Chronic fatigue immune dysfunction syndrome in 103 patients—diagnosis, test results, and therapy. Zeitschrift fur Klinische Medizin (German) 1992; 47(4):152–66.

Hodson AD. Myalgic encephalomyelitis. J Roy Soc Med 1990; 83.

Holborow PL. The ME syndrome [letter]. NZ Med J 14 Dec 1988; 835.

Holland R. Chronic fatigue syndrome [letter]. Can Med Assoc J May 1989; 140(9):1016.

Holmes GP. Defining the chronic fatigue syndrome. Rev Inf Dis 1991a; 13(Suppl 1):S53–5.

Holmes GP. The chronic fatigue syndrome. Current Opin in Inf Dis 1991b; 4:615–20.

Holmes GP. Recent developments in the chronic fatigue syndrome. Current Opin in Inf Dis 1992; 5:647–53.

Holmes GP, Kaplan JE, Gantz NM, Komaroff AL, Schonberger LB, Straus SE, et al. Chronic fatigue syndrome: a working case definition. Ann Intern Med 1988; 108:387–9.

Holmes GP, Kaplan JE, Stewart JA, Hunt B, Pinsky PF, Schonberger LB. A cluster of patients with a chronic mononucleosis-like syndrome. Is Epstein-Barr virus the cause? JAMA 1987; 257:2297–302.

Horrobin D. Post viral fatigue syndrome, viral infections in atopic excema and essential fatty acids. Medical Hypotheses 1990; 32:211–17.

Hotchin NA, Read R, Smith DG, Crawford DH. Active Epstein-Barr virus infection in post-viral fatigue syndrome. J Infect 1989; 18(2):143–50.

Howard JM, Davies S, Hunnisett A. Magnesium and chronic fatigue syndrome. Lancet 1992; 340:426.

Ho-Yen DO. Patient management of post-viral fatigue syndrome. Br J Gen Pract 1990a; 40(330):37-9.

Ho-Yen DO. Patient management and the post-viral fatigue syndrome. Br J Gen Pract 1990b; 40:(331):82-3.

Ho-Yen DO. The epidemiology of post viral fatigue syndrome. Scott Med J Dec 1988; 33(6):368-9.

Ho-Yen DO, Billington RW, Urquhart J. Natural killer cells and the post viral fatigue syndrome. Scand J of Inf Dis 1991; 23:711-6.

Ho-Yen DO, Carrington D, Armstrong AA. Myalgic encephalomyelitis and alpha interferon [letter]. Lancet 16 Jan 1988; 125.

Huang A, Quinlan AV. The post-infectious chronic fatigue syndrome: measurement of disability. *In* Epstein-Barr virus and human disease, eds Ablashi DV et al, Humana Press, 1989; 429-32.

Hudson JI, Pope HG. Chronic fatigue syndrome [letter]. JAMA 1991; 265:357-8.

Hyde B. Myalgic encephalomyelitis, Nightingale Research Foundation, Ottawa, Canada, 1989.

Hyde B, Bergmann S. Akureyri disease (myalgic encephalomyelitis) forty years later. Lancet 1988; ii:1191-2531.

Hyde BM, Goldstein J, Levine P, eds. The clinical and scientific basis of myalgic encephalomyelitis / chronic fatigue syndrome, Nightingale Research Foundation, Ottawa, Canada, 1992.

Ichise M, Salit IE, Abbey SE, Chung DG, Gray B, Kirsh JC, Freedman M. Assessment of regional cerebral perfusion by 99Tcm-HMPAO SPECT in chronic fatigue syndrome. Nuclear Medicine Communications 1992; 13(10):767-72.

Jackson JA. Chronic fatigue [letter]. JAMA 1989; 261:696.

Jagannath P. Myalgic encephalomyelitis [letter]. The Practitioner 1990; 234:326.

Jamal GA, Hansen S. Electrophysiological studies in the post viral fatigue syndrome. J Neurol, Neurosurg and Psychiat 1985; 48:691-4.

Jamal GA, Hansen S. Post viral fatigue syndrome: evidence for underlying organic disturbance in muscle fiber. Eur Neurol 1989; 2(4):427-32.

James DG, Brook MG, Bannister B. The chronic fatigue syndrome. Postgraduate Medical J 1992; 68:611-4.

Janus T. Chronic fatigue syndrome [letter]. JAMA 1991; 265:358.

Joncas JH, Ghibu F, Blagdon M, Montplaisir S, Stefanescu I, Menezes J. A familial syndrome of susceptibility to chronic active Epstein-Barr virus infection. Can Med Assoc J 1984; 130:280-5.

Jones J, Streib J, Baker S, Herberger M. Chronic fatigue syndrome: EBV immune response and molecular epidemiology. J Med Virology 1991; 33:151-8.

Jones JF. The Epstein-Barr "chronic fatigue" syndrome: evaluation guidelines. Female Patient 1988a; 13:60-7.

Jones JF. Chronic Epstein-Barr virus syndrome. Bull NY Acad Med Jul–Aug 1988b; 64(6):538-43.

Jones JF. The post-infectious chronic fatigue syndrome: management of PICFS. *In* Epstein-Barr virus and human disease, eds Ablashi DV et al, Humana Press, 1989; 432-4.

Jones JF. Serologic and immunologic responses in chronic fatigue syndrome with emphasis on the Epstein-Barr virus. Rev Inf Dis 1991; 13(Suppl 1):S26-31.

Jones JF, Shurin S, Abramowsky C, et al. T-cell lymphomas containing Epstein-Barr viral DNA in patients with chronic Epstein-Barr virus infections. N Eng J Med 1988; 318:733-41.

Jones JF, Williams M, Schooley RT, Robinson C, Glaser R. Antibodies to Epstein-Barr virus—specific DNase and DNA polymerase in the chronic fatigue syndrome. Arch Intern Med 1988; 148:1957-60.

Jones JJ, Ray CG, Minnich LL, Hicks MJ, Kibler R, Lucas DO. Evidence for active Epstein-Barr virus infection in patients with persistent, unexplained illnesses: elevated anti-early antigen antibodies. Ann Intern Med 1985; 102:1-6.

Jones JJ, Straus SE. Chronic Epstein-Barr virus infection. Ann Rev Med 1987; 38:195-206.

Josephs SF, Henry B, Balachandran N, Strayer D, Peterson D, Komaroff AL. HHV-6 reactivation in chronic fatigue syndrome [letter]. Lancet 1991; 337:1346-7.

Kaplan M. The post-infectious chronic fatigue syndrome: diagnosis in adults. *In* Epstein-Barr virus and human disease, eds Ablashi DV et al, Humana Press, 1989; 408-12.

Kaslow JE, Rucker L, Onishi R. Liver extract-folic acid-cyanocobalamin vs placebo for chronic fatigue syndrome. Arch Int Med 1989; 149:2501-3.

Katon W, Russo J. Chronic fatigue syndrome criteria—a critique of the requirements for multiple physical complaints. Arch Intern Med 1992; 152:1604-9.

Katon WJ, Buchwald DS, Simon GE, Russo JE, Mease PJ. Psychiatric illness in chronic fatigue syndrome. J Gen Int Med 1991; 6(4):277-85.

Katz BZ, Andiman WA. Progressive and chronic Epstein-Barr virus infection. Mediguide to Infectious Disease 1986; 6:1-5.

Katz BZ, Andiman WA. Chronic fatigue syndrome. J Peds 1988; 113:944-7.

Kaufman RE: Recurrences in infectious mononucleosis. Am Prac 1950; 1:673-6.

Kawai K, Kawai A. Studies on the relationship between chronic fatigue syndrome and Epstein-Barr virus in Japan. Internal Medicine 1992; 31(3):313-8.

Kendall RE. Chronic fatigue, viruses and depression. Lancet 1991; 337:160-2.

Kennedy HG. Fatigue and fatigability [letter]. Lancet 1987; i:1145.

Khan AS, Heneine WM, Chapman LE, Gary HE, Woods TC, Folks TM, Schonberger LB. Assessment of a retrovirus sequence and other possible risk factors for the chronic fatigue syndrome in adults. Ann Intern Med 1993; 118:241-5.

Kibler R, Lucas DO, Hicks MJ, Poulos BT, Jones JF. Immune function in chronic active Epstein-Barr virus infection. J Clin Immunol 1985; 5:46-54.

Klein E, Masucci MG. Cell mediated immunity against Epstein-Barr virus infected B lymphocytes. Springer Semin Immunopathol 1982; 5:63-73.

Klimas NG, Salvato FR, Morgan R, Fletcher MA. Immunologic abnormalities in the chronic fatigue syndrome. J Clin Microbiol 1990; 28:1403-10.

Klonoff DC. Chronic fatigue syndrome. CID 1992; 15(5):812-23.

Komaroff A. The "chronic mononucleosis" syndromes. Hosp Pract 1987; 71-75.

Komaroff A. HHV-6 and human disease. Am J Clin Path 1990; 93(6):836-7.

Komaroff A, Goldenberg D. The chronic fatigue syndrome: definition, current studies and lessons for fibromyalgia research. J Rheumatol Suppl 1989; 19:23-7.

Komaroff AL. Chronic fatigue syndromes: relationship to chronic viral infections. J Virol Methods 1988; 21:3-10.

Komaroff AL, Buchwald D. Symptoms and signs of chronic fatigue syndrome. Rev Inf Dis 1991; 13(Suppl 1):S9-12.

Komaroff AL, Geiger AM, Wormseley S. IgG subclass deficiencies in chronic fatigue syndrome. Lancet 1988; i(8597):1288-9.

Komaroff AL, Straus SE, Gantz NM, Jones JF. The chronic fatigue syndrome [letter]. Ann Intern Med 1989; 110:407-8.

Koo D. Chronic fatigue syndrome. A critical appraisal of the role of Epstein-Barr virus. West Med J 1989; 150(5):590-6.

Kreuger G. The post-infectious chronic fatigue syndrome: a historical perspective. *In* Epstein-Barr virus and human disease, eds Ablashi DV et al, Humana Press, 1989; 407-8.

Kreuger GRF, Koch B, Ablashi D. Persistent fatigue and depression in patient with antibody to human B-lymphotropic virus. Lancet 1987; ii:36.

Kroenke K. Chronic fatigue [letter]. JAMA 1989; 261:697.

Kroenke K. Chronic fatigue syndrome: is it real? Postgrad Med 1991; 89(2):44-6, 49-50, 53-5.

Kroenke K, Wood DR, Mangelsedorff D, Meier NJ, Powell JB. Chronic fatigue in primary care, prevalence, patient characteristics and outcome. JAMA 1988; 260:929-34.

Kruesi MJP, Dale J, Straus SE. Psychiatric diagnoses in patients who have chronic fatigue syndrome. J Clin Psychiatry 1989; 50:2 53-56.

Krupp LB, LaRocca NG, Muir-Nash J, Steinberg AD. The fatigue severity scale. Arch Neurol 1989; 46:1121-3.

Krupp LB, Mendelson WB, Friedman R. An overview of chronic fatigue syndrome. J Clin Psychiatry 1991; 52:403-10.

Kulig JW. Chronic fatigue syndrome and fibromyalgia in adolescence. Adolescent Medicine: State of the Art Reviews 1991; 2:473-84.

Kuratsune H, Yamaguti K, Takahashi M, Misaki H, Kitani T. Acylcarnitine deficiency in chronic fatigue syndrome [abstract]. Proceedings 1st International CFS/ME Conference, Albany, NY, 1-3 October 1992.

Kuwano K, Arai S, Munakata T, Tomita Y, Yoshitake Y, Kumagai K. Suppressive effect of human natural killer cells on Epstein-Barr virus-induced immunoglobulin synthesis. J Immunol 1986; 137:1462-7.

Kyle DV, deShazo RD. Chronic fatigue syndrome: a conundrum. Am J Med Sci 1992; 303(1):28-34.

Landay AL, Jessop C, Lennette ET, Levy JA. Chronic fatigue syndrome: clinical condition associated with immune activation. Lancet 1991; 338(8769); 707-12.

Lane TJ, Manu P, Matthews DA. Prospective diagnostic evaluation of adults with chronic fatigue [abstract]. Clin Res 1988; 36:714A.

Lane TJ, Manu P, Matthews DA. Depression and somatization in the chronic fatigue syndrome. Am J Med 1991; 91:335-44.

Lane TJ, Matthews DA, Manu P. The low yield of physical examinations and laboratory investigations of patients with chronic fatigue. Am J Med Sci 1990; 299(5):313-8.

Lapp CW. Chronic fatigue syndrome is a real disease. North Carolina Family Physician 1992; 43:6-9.

Lask B, Dillon MJ. Postviral fatigue syndrome. Arch Dis Child 1990; 65(11):1198.

Lasky HP. Chronic EBV infection and PMR [letter]. J Rheumatol Mar 1989; 16(3): 414-5.

Lechky O. Life insurance MDs sceptical when chronic fatigue syndrome diagnosed. Can Med Assoc J 1990; 143:413-5.

Lehrer JF, Hover LM. Fatigue syndrome [letter]. JAMA 1988; 259:842-3.

Lev M. Myalgic encephalomyelitis [letter]. J Roy Soc Med 1989; 82(11):693-4.

Lever AML, Lewis DM, Bannister BA, Fry M, Berry N. Interferon production in postviral fatigue syndrome. Lancet 9 July 1988; 101.

Levine P. The post-infectious chronic fatigue syndrome: concluding remarks. *In* Epstein-Barr virus and human disease, eds Ablashi DV et al, Humana Press, 1989; 434-8.

Levine PH, Jacobson S, Pocinki AG, Cheney P, Peterson D, Connelley RR, Weil R, Robinson SM, Ablashi D, Salahuddin SZ, Pearson GR, Hoover R. Clinical, epidemiologic, and virologic studies in four clusters of the chronic fatigue syndrome. Arch Int Med 1992; 152:1611-6.

Lewis SF, Haller RG. Physiologic measurement of exercise and fatigue with special reference to chronic fatigue syndrome. Rev Inf Dis 1991; 13(Suppl 1):S98-108.

Leyton E, Pross H. Chronic fatigue syndrome. Do herbs or homeopathy help? Can Family Physician 1992; 38:2021-6.

Lieberman J. Angiotensin-converting enzyme in nonpulmonary sarcoidosis. Sem in Resp Medicine 1992; 13(5):399-401.

Lieberman J, Bell DS. Serum angiotensin converting enzyme (SACE): a diagnostic aid for chronic fatigue syndrome. Clin Res 1991; 39:129A.

Linde A, Andersson B, Svenson SB, Ahrne H, Carlsson M, Forsberg P, Hugo H, Karstorp A, Lenkei R, Lindwall A, Loftenius A, Sall C, Andersson J. Serum levels of lymphokines and soluble cellular receptors in primary Epstein-Barr virus infection and in patients with chronic fatigue syndrome. J Inf Dis 1992; 165 (6):994-1000.

Linde A, Hammarstrom L, Smith CIE. IgG subclass deficiency and chronic fatigue syndrome. Lancet 1988; 8590:885-6.

Littlejohn GO, Weinstein C, Helme RD. Increased neurogenic inflammation in fibrositis syndrome. J Rheumatol 1987; 14:1022-5.

Lloyd A. Muscle vs brain: chronic fatigue syndrome. Med J Aust 1990; 153:530-4.

Lloyd A, Hanna DA, Wakefield D. Interferon and myalgic encephalomyelitis. Lancet 1988; i(8583):471.

Lloyd A, Hickie I, Boughton CR, Spencer O, Wakefield D. Prevalence of chronic fatigue syndrome in an Australian population. Med J Aust 1990; 153:522-8.

Lloyd A, Hickie I, Brockman A, Dwyer J, Wakefield D. Cytokine levels in serum and cerebrospinal fluid in patients with chronic fatigue syndrome and control subjects. J Inf Dis 1991; 199:164.

Lloyd A, Hickie I, Hickie C, Dwyer J, Wakefield D. Cell-mediated immunity in patients with chronic fatigue syndrome, healthy control subjects, and patients with major depression. Clin Exp Immunol 1992; 87:76-9.

Lloyd A, Hickie I, Wakefield D. Immunological abnormalities in the chronic fatigue syndrome [letter]. Med J Aust 1990; 152:51.

Lloyd A, Hickie I, Wakefield D, Boughton C, Dwyer J. A double-blind, placebo-controlled trial of intravenous immunoglobulin therapy in patients with chronic fatigue syndrome. Am J Med 1990; 89:561-8.

Lloyd AR, Gandevia SC, Hales JP. Muscle performance, voluntary activation, twitch properties, and perceived effort in normal subjects and patients with the chronic fatigue syndrome. Brain 1991; 114:85-98.

Lloyd AR, Wakefield D, Boughton C, Dwyer J. What is myalgic encephalomyelitis? Lancet 1988; i(8597):1286–7.

Lloyd AR, Wakefield D, Boughton CR, Dwyer JM. Immunological abnormalities in the chronic fatigue syndrome. Med J Aust 1989; 151(3):122–4.

Luca J, Okana M, Thiele G. Isolation of human herpes virus-6 from clinical specimens using human fibroblast cultures. J Clin Lab Analysis 1990; 4(6):483–6.

Lynch S, Main J, Seth R. Definition of the chronic fatigue syndrome. Brit J Psychiat 1991; 159:439–40.

Lynch S, Seth R. Postviral fatigue syndrome and the VP-1 Antigen. Lancet 1989; ii:1160–1.

Lynch S, Seth R. Depression and myalgic encephalomyelitis [letter]. J Roy Soc Med 1990; 83(6):413.

Lynch SPJ, Seth RV, Main J. Monospot and VP1 tests in chronic fatigue syndrome and major depression. J Roy Soc Med 1992; 85:537–40.

Mangi RJ, Niederman JC, Kelleher JE, Dwyer JM, Evans AS, Kantor FS. Depression of cell mediated immunity during acute infectious mononucleosis. N Eng J Med 1974; 291:1149–53.

Manu P, et al. Depression among patients with a complaint of chronic fatigue. J Affect Disord 1989; 17(2):165–72.

Manu P, Lane TJ, Matthews DA. The frequency of chronic fatigue syndrome in patients with persistent fatigue. Ann Intern Med 1988; 109:554–6.

Marshall GS, Gesser RM, Yamanishi K, Starr SE. Chronic fatigue in children: clinical features, Epstein-Barr virus and human herpes virus 6 serology and long term follow-up. Ped Inf Dis 1991; 10:287–90.

Matthews DA, Manu P, Lane TJ. Evaluation and management of patients with chronic fatigue. Am J Med Sci 1991; 302:269.

May PBR, Donnan SPB, Ashton JR, Ogilvie MM, Rolles CJ. Personality and medical perception in benign myalgic encephalomyelitis. Lancet 1980; ii:1122–4.

McBride SJ, McClusky DR. Treatment of chronic fatigue syndrome. Br Med Bull 1991; 47(4):895–907.

McCain G. Toward an understanding of FM syndrome. Pain 1991; 45:227–48.

McClusky D. Aerobic work capacity in patients with chronic fatigue syndrome. BMJ 1990; 301:956–61.

McEvedy CP, Beard AW. Concept of benign myalgic encephalomyelitis. Br Med J 1970a; i:11–5.

McEvedy CP, Beard AW. Royal Free epidemic of 1955: a reconsideration. Br Med J 1970b; 1:7–11.

Medical Staff of the Royal Free Hospital. An outbreak of encephalomyelitis in the Royal Free Hospital Group, London, in 1955. Br Med J 1957; 2:895–904.

Meth RJ. Chronic fatigue [letter]. JAMA 1989; 261:696-7.

Middleton D, Savage DA, Smith DG. No association of HLA class II antigens in chronic fatigue syndrome. Disease Markers 1991; 9:47-9.

Miller G. Molecular approaches to epidemiologic evaluation of viruses as risk factors for patients who have chronic fatigue syndrome. Rev Inf Dis 1991; 13(Suppl 1):S119-22.

Miller G, Grogan E, Rowe D, Rooney C, Heston L, Eastman R, et al. Selective lack of antibody to a component of EB nuclear antigen in patients with chronic active Epstein-Barr virus infection. J Inf Dis 1987; 156:26-35.

Miller NA, Carmichael HA, Calder BD, Behan PO, Bell EJ, McCartney RA, Hall FC. Antibody to Coxsackie B virus in diagnosing postviral fatigue syndrome. BMJ 1991; 302(6769):140-3.

Moldofsky H. Sleep and fibrositis syndrome. Rheum Clin NA 1989a; 15:91-103.

Moldofsky H. Non-restorative sleep and symptoms after a febrile illness in patients with fibrositis and chronic fatigue syndromes. J Rheumatol Suppl 1989b; 19: 150-3.

Moldofsky H, Saskin P, Lue FA. Sleep and symptoms in fibrositis syndrome after a febrile illness. J Rheumatol 1988; 15:1701-4.

Montague TJ, Marrie TJ, Klassen GA, Bewick DJ, Horacek BM. Cardiac function at rest and with exercise in the chronic fatigue syndrome. Chest Apr 1989; 95(4):779-84.

Morag A, Tobi M, Ravid Z, et al. Lancet 1982; 744.

Morrison LJA, Behan WHM, Behan PO. Changes in natural cell phenotype in patients with post-viral fatigue syndrome. Clin Exp Immunol 1991; 83:441-6.

Morte S, Castilla A, Iveira MP, Serrano M, Prieto J. Production of Interleukin-1 by peripheral blood mononuclear cells in patients with chronic fatigue syndrome [letter]. J Inf Dis 1989; 159:362.

Moss DJ, Misko IS, et al. J Exp Clin Cancer Res (Supplement) 1988; 7, 57.

Mowbray JF, Yousef GE. Immunology of the post viral fatigue syndrome. Br Med Bull 1991; 47(4):886-94.

Mukherjee TM, Smith K, Maros K. Abnormal red-blood-cell morphology in myalgic encephalomyelitis. Lancet 1987.

Murdoch JC. Myalgic encephalomyelitis and the general practitioner. NZ Family Phys 1984; 11:127-8.

Murdoch JC. Myalgic encephalomyelitis (ME) syndrome—an analysis of the clinical findings in 200 cases. NZ Family Phys 1987a; 14:51-4.

Murdoch JC. Post-viral syndrome [letter]. J Roy Col Gen Pract 1987b; 512.

Murdoch JC. Cell-mediated immunity in patients with myalgic encephalomyelitis syndrome. NZ Med J 1988; 101:511-2.

Murray JB. Psychological aspects of chronic fatigue syndrome. Perceptual and Motor Skills 1992; 74:1123–36.

Myalgic Encephalomyelitis Association. Guidelines for parents of children with ME. PO Box 8, Stanford-le-hope, Essex, England, SS17 8EX; 1989.

Newsholme EA, Blomstrand E, Hassmen P, Ekblom B. Physical and mental fatigue: do changes in plasma amino acids play a role? Biochemical Society Transactions, Vol 19, 1991; 362–7.

Niederman JC. Chronicity of Epstein-Barr virus infection [editorial]. Ann Intern Med 1985; 102:119–20.

Nielsen J. Immunological abnormalities in the chronic fatigue syndrome [letter]. Med J Aust 1990; 152:51.

Office of Communications, National Institute of Allergy and Infectious Diseases. Backgrounder: chronic fatigue syndrome, National Institutes of Health, June 1988.

Okano M, Thiele GM, Davis JR, Nauseef WM, Mitros F, Purtilo DT. Adenovirus type-2 in a patient with lethal hemorrhagic colonic ulcers and chronic active Epstein-Barr virus infection. Ann Intern Med 1988; 108:693–9.

Olson GB, Kanaan MN, Gersuk GM, Kelley LM, Jones JF. Correlation between allergy and persistent Epstein-Barr virus infection in chronic-active Epstein-Barr virus infected patients. J Allergy Clin Immunol 1986; 78:308–14.

Olson GB, Kanaan MS, Kelley LM, Jones JF. Specific allergen-induced Epstein-Barr nuclear antigen-positive B cells from patients with chronic active Epstein-Barr virus infections. J Allergy Clin Immunol 1986, 78:315–20.

Palca J. Does a retrovirus explain fatigue syndrome puzzle? Science 1990; 249(4974):1240–1.

Palca J. On the track of an elusive disease. Science 1992; 254:1726–7.

Pamphlett R, Odonoghue P. Antibodies against sarcocystis and toxoplasma in humans with chronic fatigue syndrome. Australian and New Zealand Journal of Medicine 1992; 22(3):307.

Parish JG. Epidemic neuromyasthenia: a reappraisal. Journal of International Research Communications in Medical Sciences 1974; 2:22–6.

Parish JG. Early outbreaks of "epidemic neuromyasthenia." Postgraduate Med J 1978; 54:711–7.

Patterson JK, Pinninger JL. A case of recurrent infectious mononucleosis. Br Med J 1955; 32:246.

Payne CB, Sloan HE. Pulmonary function and the chronic fatigue syndrome. Ann Intern Med 1989; 111:860.

Peel M. Rehabilitation in postviral syndrome. J Soc Occup Med 1988; 38:44–5.

Pellegrino MJ, Waylonis GW, Sommer A. Familial occurrence of primary fibro-myalgia. Arch Phys Med Rehabil 1989; 70:61-3.

Pellew RAA. A clinical description of a disease resembling poliomyelitis, seen in Adelaide, 1949-1951. Med J Aust June 1951; 944-6.

Pelosi AJ, David AS. Postviral fatigue syndrome. BMJ 1988; 296:1329-30.

Perrins DJD. The diagnosis of postviral syndrome. J Roy Soc Med 1990; 83:413.

Peterson D, Cheney P, Ford M, Hunt B, Reynolds G. Chronic fatigue possibly related to Epstein-Barr virus Nevada. MMWR 1986; 35:350-2.

Peterson PK, Shepard J, Macres M, Schenck C, Crosson J, Rechtman D, Lurie N. A controlled trial of intravenous immunoglobulin G in chronic fatigue syndrome. Am J Med 1990; 89(5):554-60.

Poore M, Snow P, Paul C. An unexplained illness in West Otago. NZ Med J 1984; 97:351-4.

Poskanzer DC, Henderson DA, Kunkle EC, Kalter SS, Clement WB, Bond JO. Epidemic neuromyasthenia: an outbreak in Punta Gorda, Florida. N Eng J Med 1957; 257:356-64.

Potaznick W, Kozol N. Ocular manifestations of chronic fatigue and immune dys-function syndrome. Optometry and Visual Science 1992; 69:811-4.

Powell MA. Epstein-Barr antibody and chronic fatigue syndrome. J Am Acad Nurse Pract 1990; 2(1):33-4.

Powell S. Myalgic encephalomyelitis [letter]. Br J Gen Pract 1990; 40(333):170.

Prasher D, Smith A, Findley L. Sensory and cognitive event-related potentials in myalgic encephalomyelitis. J Neurol Neurosurg Psychiatry 1990; 53(3):247-53.

Price RK, North CS, Wessely S, Fraser VJ. Estimating the prevalence of chronic fatigue syndrome and associated symptoms in the community. Public Health Reports 1992; 107(5):514-22.

Prieto J, Subir'a ML, Castilla A, Serrano M. Naloxone reversible monocyte dys-function in patients with chronic fatigue syndrome. Scand J Immunol 1989; 30(1):13-20.

Pritchard C. Fibrositis and the chronic fatigue syndrome [letter]. Ann Intern Med 1988; 106:906.

Purtilo DT, Sakomoto K. Epstein-Barr virus and human disease immune responses determine the clinical and pathologic expression. Hum Path 1981; 12:677-9.

Purvan Z. Postviral syndrome [letter]. Med J Aust 1987; 147:524.

Ramsay M. Myalgic encephalomyelitis: a baffling syndrome. Nursing Mirror Oct 1981; 40-1.

Ramsay MA. Postviral fatigue syndrome: the saga of Royal Free disease. Gower Medical Publishing, London, 1986.

Ramsay MA. Myalgic encephalitis and postviral fatigue states: the saga of Royal Free disease. Second Edition. Gower Medical Publishing, London, 1988.

Ray C, Weir WRC, Phillips S, Cullen S. Development of a measure of symptoms in chronic fatigue syndrome: the profile of fatigue-related symptoms (PFRS). Psychology and Health 1992; 7:27–43.

Read R, Spickett G, Harvey J, Edwards AJ, Larson HE. IgG1 subclass deficiency in patients with chronic fatigue syndrome. Lancet 1988; i:241–2.

Redmond CK. Analysis of clinical, epidemiologic, and laboratory data on chronic fatigue syndrome. Rev Inf Dis 1991; 13(Suppl 1):S90–3.

Reeves WC, Pellett PE, Gary H. The chronic fatigue syndrome controversy [letter]. Ann Intern Med 1992; 117:343.

Reilly PA, Littlejohn GO. Fibromyalgia and chronic fatigue syndrome. Cur Opinion Rheum 1990; 2(2):282–90.

Reiss GR. The Epstein-Barr virus and chronic fatigue syndrome [letter]. 1989; 261:1287.

Reiss GR. Chronic fatigue syndrome [letter]. J Clin Psychiat 1990; 51(4):169.

Renfro L, Feder HM, Lane TJ, Manu P, Matthews DA. Yeast connection among 100 patients with chronic fatigue. Am J Med 1989; 86:165–8.

Riccio M, Thompson C, Wilson B, Morgan DJR, Lant AF. Neuropsychological and psychiatric abnormalities in myalgic encephalomyelitis: a preliminary report. British J of Clin Psychology 1992; 31:111–20.

Risdale L. Chronic fatigue in a family practice. J Fam Pract 1989; 29(5):486–8.

Romano TJ. Fibromyalgia in children; diagnosis and treatment. W Va Med J 1991; 87:112–4.

Rose E, Jagannath P, Wessely S. Possible ME. Practitioner 1990; 234(1484):195–8.

Rosen SD, King JC, Nixon PGF. Myalgic encephalomyelitis. J Roy Soc Med 1990: 83.

Rosen SD, King JC, Wilkinson JB, Nixon PG. Is chronic fatigue syndrome synonymous with effort syndrome? J Roy Soc Med 1990; 83(12):761–4.

Ross GH, Rea WJ, Johnson AR. Chronic fatigue syndrome [letter]. Can Med Assoc J 1989; 141(1):11–2.

Rutherford OM, White PD. Human quadriceps strength and fatigability in patients with post viral fatigue. J Neurol, Neurosurg and Psychiat 1991; 54(11):961–4.

Salit I. Understanding the chronic fatigue syndrome. Canadian Journal of Diagnosis 1992; 9:52–65.

Salit IE. Sporadic postinfectious neuromyasthenia. Can Med Assoc J 1985; 133: 659–63.

Salvato F, Fletcher M, Ashman M, Klimas N. Immune dysfunction among chronic fatigue syndrome (CFS) patients with clear evidence of Epstein-Barr virus (EBV) reactivation. J Exp Clin Cancer Res (suppl) 1988; 7(3):89.

Scheffers MK, Johnson R, Grafman J, Dale JK, Straus SE. Attention and short term memory in chronic fatigue syndrome patients: an event-related potential analysis. Neurology 1992; 42:1667-75.

Schluederberg A, Straus S, Perterson P, Blumenthal S, Komaroff AL, Spring SB, Landay A, Buchwald D. Chronic fatigue syndrome research: Definition and medical outcome assessment. NIH Conference. Ann Intern Med 1992; 117: 325-31.

Schooley RT. Chronic fatigue syndrome: A manifestation of Epstein-Barr virus infection? *In* Current clinical topics in infectious diseases, No 9, eds Remington J, Swatz MN, McGraw-Hill, New York; 1988; 126-46.

Schulte PA. Validation of biologic markers for use in research on chronic fatigue syndrome. Rev Inf Dis 1991; 13(Suppl 1):S87-9.

Schwartz DL, Bottom WD. Chronic fatigue syndrome: an epidemiologic and diagnostic enigma. J Am Acad Phys Assist 1989; 2:176-82.

Shafran S. The chronic fatigue syndrome. Amer J Med 1991; 90:730-9.

Sharpe MC, Archard LC, Banatvala JE, Boryseiwicz LK, Clare AW, David A, et al. A report—chronic fatigue syndrome: guidelines for research. J R Soc Med 1991; 84:118-21.

Sharpe MC, Johnson BA, McCann J. Mania and recovery from chronic fatigue syndrome. J Roy Soc Med 1991; 84(1):51-2.

Shelokov A, Habel K, Verder E, Welsh W. Epidemic neuromyasthenia: an outbreak of poliomyelitislike illness in student nurses. N Eng J Med 1957; 257:345-55.

Shepherd C. How I treat myalgic encephalomyelitis: forum [letter]. The Practitioner 1990; 234(1486):326.

Sherry DD, McGuire T, Mellins E, Salsmonson K, Wallace CA, Nepom B. Psychosomatic musculoskeletal pain in childhood: clinical and psychological analyses of 100 children. Pediatrics 1992; 88:1093-9.

Shore A, Klock R, Lee P, Snow KM, Keystone EC. Impaired late suppression of Epstein-Barr virus (EBV)-induced immunoglobulin synthesis: a common feature of autoimmune disease. J Clin Immunol 1989; 9(2):103-10.

Sigler AT. Chronic fatigue syndrome: fact or fiction? Contemporary Pediatrics 1990; 7:22-50.

Sigurdsson B, Sigurjonsson J, Sigurdsson JH, Thorkelsson J, Gudmundsson KR. A disease epidemic in Iceland simulating poliomyelitis. Am J Hyg 1950; 52:222-38.

Simpson LO. Are ME and chronic fatigue syndrome the same? [letter]. NZ Med J 1990; 103(892):305.

Simpson LO. Nondiscocytic erythrocytes in myalgic encephalomyelitis. NZ Med J 1989; 102(864):126-7.

Simpson LO. Myalgic encephalomyelitis [letter]. J Roy Soc Med 1991; 84:633.

Simpson LO, Shand BI, Olds RJ. Blood rheology and myalgic encephalomyelitis. Pathology 1986; 18:190–2.

Singer A, Thompson S, Kraiuhin C, Gordon E, Howe G, Howson A, Meares R. An investigation of patients presenting with multiple physical complaints using the illness behaviour questionnaire. Psychother Psychosom 1987; 47:181–9.

Smith AP. Chronic fatigue syndrome and performance. *In* Handbook of human performance, Vol 2; eds Smith AP, Jones D, Academic Press, London, 1992; 261–78.

Smith D. Some guidelines on the education of children. Myalgic Encephalomyelitis Association, 1989.

Smith H, Denman AM. A new manifestation of infection with Epstein-Barr virus. Br Med J Clin Res 1978; 2:248.

Smith MS, Mitchell J, Corey L, Gold D, McCauley EA, Glover D, Tenover FC. Chronic fatigue in adolescents. Pediatrics 1991; 88(2):195–202.

Straus S. The chronic mononucleosis syndrome. J Inf Dis 1988; 157:405–12.

Straus S. Chronic fatigue syndrome: a troubling dilemma. PA Pract 1989; 8:14–6.

Straus S. History of chronic fatigue syndrome. Rev Inf Dis 1991; 13(Suppl 1):S2–8.

Straus SE. EB or not EB—That is the question [editorial]. JAMA 1987; 257:2335–6.

Straus SE. Intravenous gammaglobulin treatment for the chronic fatigue syndrome. Am J Med 1990; 89(5):551–3.

Straus SE. Defining the chronic fatigue syndrome. Arch Intern Med 1992; 152: 1569–70.

Straus SE, Dale JK, Peter JB, Dinarello CA. Circulating lymphokine levels in the chronic fatigue syndrome [letter]. J Infect Dis 1989; 160(6):1085–6.

Straus SE, Dale JK, Tobi M, Lawley T, Preble O, Blaese RM, Hallahan C, Henle W. Acyclovir treatment of the chronic fatigue syndrome. N Eng J Med 1988; 319:1692–8.

Straus SE, Tosato G, Armstrong G, Lawley T, Preble OT, Henle W, Davey R, Pearson G, Epstein J, Brus I, Blaese M. Persisting illness and fatigue in adults with evidence of Epstein-Barr virus infection. Ann Intern Med 1985; 102:7–16.

Strayer D, Gillespie D, Peterson D, Cheney P, Salvato P, Loveless M, Fletcher M, Klimas N, Patarca R, Suhadolnik R, Walters D, Carter W. Treatment of chronic fatigue immune dysfunction syndrome with Poly (I):Poly(C12U). Presented at the 31st ICAAC Meetings, Chicago, 1 Oct 1991.

Strickland MC. Depression, chronic fatigue syndrome and the adolescent. Primary Care 1991; 18:259–70.

Stricklin A, Sewell M, Austad C. Objective measurement of personality variables in epidemic neuromyasthenia patients. S Afr Med J 1990; 77(1):31–4.

Sturtz GS. Depression and chronic fatigue in children. Primary Care 1991; 18: 247–57.

Subir'a ML, Castilla A, Civeira MP, Prieto J. Deficient display of CD3 on lymphocytes of patients with chronic fatigue syndrome [letter]. J Infect Dis July 1989; 160(1):165–6.

Sumaya CV. Endogenous reactivation of Epstein-Barr virus infections. J Infect Dis 1977; 135:374–9.

Sumaya CV. Infectious mononucleosis and other Epstein-Barr infections: diagnostic factors. Lab Management 1986; 37–42.

Sumaya CV. Serologic and virologic epidemiology of Epstein-Barr virus: relevance to chronic fatigue syndrome. Rev Inf Dis 1991; 13(Suppl 1):S19–25.

Sumner DW. Further outbreak of a disease resembling poliomyelitis. Lancet 1956; i:764–6.

Swartz MN. The chronic fatigue syndrome—one entity or many? [editorial]. N Eng J Med 1988; 319:1726–8.

Thase ME. Assessment of depression in chronic fatigue syndrome. Rev Inf Dis 1991; 13(Suppl 1):S114–8.

Thomas PK. Postviral fatigue syndrome. Lancet 24 Jan 1987; 218–9.

Tobi M, Morag A, Ravid Z, Chowers I, Feldman-Weiss Y, Michaeli Y, Ben-Chetrit E, Shalit M, Knobler H. Prolonged atypical illness associated with serologic evidence of persistent Epstein-Barr virus infection. Lancet 1982; 1:61–4.

Tobi M, Straus SE. Chronic Epstein-Barr virus disease: a workshop held by the National Institute of Allergy and Infectious Disease. Ann Intern Med 1985; 103:951–3.

Tobi M, Straus SE. Chronic mononucleosis—a legitimate diagnosis. Postgrad Med 1988; 83:69—78.

Tosato G, Straus S, Henle W, Pike SE, Blaese RM. Characteristic T cell dysfunction in patients with chronic active Epstein-Barr virus infections (chronic infectious mononucleosis). J Immunol 1985; 134:3082.

Troughton AH, Blacker R, Vivian G. 99mTC HMPAO SPECT in the chronic fatigue syndrome [abstract]. Clinical Radiology 1992; 45:59.

US Department of Health and Human Services. Chronic fatigue syndrome: a pamphlet for physicians. NIH Publication no. 90–484, Oct 1990.

Valdini A. Selections from the current literature: chronic fatigue syndrome. Fam Pract 1990; 7(2):152–5.

Valdini A, Steinhardt S, Feldman E. Usefulness of a standard battery of laboratory tests in investigating chronic fatigue in adults. Fam Pract 1989; 6(4):286–91.

Van Amberg RJ. Idiopathic chronic fatigue. A primary disorder. NJ Med 1990; 87(4):319–24.

Van Zelst TW. Expansion of medical research, surveillance network and public education for chronic fatigue syndrome (CFS). Statement for the record to the House Appropriations Subcommittee Labor, Health, and Human Services Education and Related Agencies, 1 May 1989.

Venables P. Epstein-Barr virus infection and autoimmunity in rheumatoid arthritis. Ann Rheum Dis 1988; 47:265–9.

Virelizier J, Lenoir G, Griscelli C. Persistent Epstein-Barr virus infection in a child with hypergammaglobulinemia and immunoblastic proliferation associated with a selective defect in immune interferon secretion. Lancet 1978; 2:231–4.

Wakefield D, Lloyd A. Pathophysiology of myalgic encephalitis. Lancet 1987; ii:918–9.

Wakefield D, Lloyd A, Brockman A. Immunoglobulin subclass abnormalities in patients with chronic fatigue syndrome. Ped Inf Dis J 1990; 9(8 Suppl):S50–3.

Wakefield D, Lloyd A, Dwyer J, Salahuddin SZ, Ablashi DV. Human herpes virus 6 and myalgic encephalomyelitis. Lancet 1988; i:1059.

Wallis AL. An investigation into an unusual disease in epidemic and sporadic form in a general practice in Cumberland in 1955 and subsequent years. University of Edinburgh doctoral thesis, 1957.

Ware N, Kleinman A. Depression in neurasthenia and chronic fatigue syndrome. Psychiatric Ann 1992a; 22(4):202–8.

Ware N, Kleinman A. Culture and somatic experience: the social course of illness in neurasthenia and chronic fatigue syndrome. Psychosomatic Med 1992b; 54(5):546–60.

Warner CL, Cookfair DL, Heffner RR, Bell DS, Ley D, Jacobs L. Neurologic abnormalities in the chronic fatigue syndrome [abstract]. Neurology 1989; 39(Suppl 1):420.

Waters-Peacocke N, Wray BB, Ades EW. A prospective study: evaluation of antibody dependent cell mediated cytotoxicity assay in chronic active Epstein-Barr syndrome. J Clin Lab Immunol Sept 1988; 27 (1):11–2.

Weinstein L. Thyroiditis and "chronic infectious mononucleosis" [letter]. JAMA 1987; 317:1225–6.

Weir WRC. The post-viral fatigue syndrome. Current Medical Literature. Infectious Diseases [Royal Society of Medicine] 1992; 6(1):3–7.

Welliver RC. Allergy and the syndrome of chronic Epstein-Barr virus infection [editorial]. J All & Clin Immunol 1986; 78(2):278–80.

Wemm KM, Trestman RL, Levine S. The effect of a laboratory stressor on natural killer cell function in chronic fatigue syndrome patients. Psychosomatics 1991; 32:470–1.

Wessely S. Myalgic encephalomyelitis—a warning: discussion paper. J R Soc Med Apr 1989; 82(4):215–7.

Wessely S. Myalgic encephalomyelitis [letter]. The Practitioner 1990a; 234:326.

Wessely S. Old wine in new bottles: neurasthenia and 'ME.' Psychol Med 1990b; 20(1):35–53.

Wessely S. History of chronic fatigue syndrome. Br Med Bull 1991; 47(4):919–41.

Wessely S. Chronic fatigue syndrome: current issues. Reviews in Medical Microbiology 1992; 3:211–6.

Wessely S, David A, Butler S, Chalder T. Manangement of post-viral syndrome [letter]. Br J Gen Pract 1990; 40(331):82–3.

Wessely S, Davis A, Pelosi A. Acyclovir treatment of the chronic fatigue syndrome [letter]. NEJM 1989; 321:187.

Wessely S, Powell R. Fatigue syndromes: a comparison of chronic "postviral" fatigue with neuromuscular and affective disorders. J Neurol Neurosurg Psychiatry 1989; 52(8); 940–8.

Wessely S, Thomas PK. The chronic fatigue syndrome (myalgic encephalomyelitis or post-viral fatigue). *In* Recent advances in neurology, Vol 6, ed Kennard C, Churchill Livingstone, Edinburgh, 1990.

Whelton CL, Salit I, Moldovsky H. Sleep, Epstein-Barr virus infection, musculo-skeletal pain and depressive symptoms in chronic fatigue syndrome. J Rheum 1992; 19:939–43.

White DN, Burtch RB. Iceland disease: a new infection simulating acute anterior poliomyelitis. Neurology 1954; 4:506–16.

Wigley RD. Chronic fatigue syndrome, ME, and fibromyalgia [letter]. NZ Med J 1990; 103:378.

Willoughby E. Myalgic encephalomyelitis [letter]. NZ Med J 25 Jan 1989; 19–20.

Wilson PM, Kusumaker V, McCartney RA, Bell EJ. Features of Coxsackie B virus (CBV) infection in children with prolonged physical and psychological morbidity. J Psychosom Res 1989; 33(1):29–36.

Winbow A. Myalgic encephalomyelitis presenting as psychiatric illness. Br J Clin & Sic Psychiat 1986; 4:29–31.

Wolfe F, Smythe HA, Yunus MA, Bennett RM, Bombardier C, Goldenberg DL, et al. The American college of rheumatology 1990 criteria for the classification of fibromyalgia. Arth & Rheum 1990; 33:160–72.

Wong KW, D'Amico DJ, Hedges TR, Soong HK, Schooley RT, Kenyon KR. Ocular involvement associated with chronic Epstein-Barr virus disease. Arch Ophthalmol 1987; 105:788–92.

Wong R, Lopaschuk G, Zhu G, Walker D, Catellier D, Burton D, Teo K, Collins-Nakai R, Montague T. Skeletal muscle metabolism in the chronic fatigue syndrome. In vivo assessment by 31P nuclear magnetic resonance spectroscopy. Chest 1992; 102(6):1716–22.

Wood GC, Bentall RP, Gopfert M, Edwards RHT. A comparative psychiatric assessment of patients with chronic fatigue syndrome and muscle disease. Psychological Med 1991; 21:619–28.

Woodward CG, Cox RA. Epstein-Barr virus serology in the chronic fatigue syndrome. J of Infection 1992; 24:133–9.

Wylie B. Muscle versus brain: chronic fatigue syndrome [letter]. Med J Aust 1991; 154(3):220.

Yousef GE, Mann GF, Smith DG, Bell EJ, Murugesan V, McCartney RA, Mowbray JF. Chronic enterovirus infection in patients with postviral fatigue syndrome. Lancet 1988; i:146–50.

Yunus MB. Aches and pains: is it juvenile fibromyalgia syndrome? Diagnosis Aug 1984; 93–102.

Yunus MB, Ahles TA, Aldag JC, Masi AT. Relationship of clinical features with psychological status in primary fibromyalgia. Arth & Rheum 1991; 34:15–21.

Yunus MB, Dailey JW, Aldag JW, Masi AT, Jobe PC. Plasma tryptophan and other amino acids in primary fibromyalgia: a controlled study. J Rheumatol 1992; 19:90–4.

Yunus MB, Masi AT. Juvenile primary fibromyalgia syndrome. Arth & Rheum 1985; 28:138–45.

Zela J. Diagnosing myalgic encephalitis. Practitioner 1989; 233(1471):916–9.

Abdomen, 41, 47
   pain in, 32, 34–35, 167
   testing of, 89–90
Ablashi, Dharam, 226
Accidents, 31
Acetaminophen, 160–61, 165, 167–68
Acetazolamide, 168
Acupuncture, 148
Acute onset of symptoms, 28, 29–31,
   139–40, 202
   in adolescents, 74
Acyclovir, 147, 170–71
Adelaide, Australia, outbreak in, 184
Adolescents, 74–75
   and cytokines, 218
Adrenal hormones, 115–16
Adrenalin symptoms, 48
   treatment of, 166, 167
Age and CFIDS, 14, 138, 140–41
"Agent X," 15, 97, 201, 210, 217–20
AIDS, 199, 204
   and autoimmunity, 99, 100
   and emotional symptoms, 59
   as nonpsychosomatic, 18
   and retrovirus, 222, 223–28
   and similarities to CFIDS, 17–18,
      87, 222–26
Akureyri, Iceland, outbreak in, 14,
   137, 183–84
Alaska, outbreak in, 137
Alertness, 164
Allergies, 15, 17, 37–38, 59–61, 62,
   154, 190, 202
   in childhood, 61
   to drugs, 159
   and immune system, 98
   treatment of, 161–62
Alpha interferon, 58
Amantadine, 166
American Cancer Society, 63
Amphetamines, 174
Ampligen, 171–72, 226

Anafranil, 165
Analgesics, 160–61
Anemia, 39
Angiotensin converting enzyme, 115
Annals of Internal Medicine, 187–88
Antibiotics, 169–70
Antibodies, 60, 87, 95–96, 227
   against Epstein-Barr virus, 107–9
   and autoimmunity, 98–99
   and retrovirus, 222
   testing for, 83
Anticoagulants, 160
Antidepressants, 163–64, 165, 166
Antihistamines, 161–62, 165
Antinuclear antibody (ANA), 88
Anxiety disorders, 37, 45, 58–59
   treatment of, 162
Aspirin, 160–61, 165, 167–68
Asthma, 38, 190, 202
Athletes, 29–30, 152
Attention problems, 44–45, 77
Atypical multiple sclerosis, 51–52
Autoimmunity, 98–99
Autonomic nervous system, 46, 48
Ayrshire, Scotland, outbreak in, 187

Bacterial infections, 31
Balance disturbance, 46, 114
Beam scan, 49
Behavior problems, 78
Bell, Karen, 190
Benedryl, 161–62
Benzodiazepines, 162, 165
Beta blockers, 167, 168
Bilirubin, 114–15
Biologic depression, 57
Blood, 208
   and spread of disease, 18
   testing of, 85, 86, 113, 114–15
Blood cells, 99–100, 211–12
Body chemicals, 58
   and immune system, 216

Bone marrow, 106
  testing of, 90
Borrelia burgdorfi, 88
Bowels
  testing of, 89–90
  treatment of, 167
Brain, 10, 47, 48, 49, 168, 208–9
  diseases of, 57, 89, 212
  and sleep, 209
  testing of, 91, 113, 114
Brain mapping, 114
Breath, 37
Breathlessness, 48
Bronchitis, 170
Brucellosis, 204
Bruising, 39
Bupropion, 164, 166
Burkitt's lymphoma, 105–6

Calcium channel blockers, 168
Camel's back theory, 206
Cancer, 63, 122, 233
  and depression, 53
  treatment of, 218
Candida, 35, 40, 95, 169, 204
  treatment of, 176
  See also Yeast
Catecholamine symptoms, 167
Cause of CFIDS, 15–18, 97, 201, 226
  as depression, 53
  testing for, 84
Cell-mediated immunity, 96, 226
Cells, 210–11
Centers for Disease Control, 7, 8,
    72, 75, 118, 131, 187
  diagnostic criteria, 26–27
Central nervous system, 44
CFIDS disability scale, 122–24
Chemical sensitivities, 31, 38, 59, 62
Chemicals of the body, 58
Chemistries, 86
Cheney, Paul, 101, 105, 187
Chest, 41, 167
Children, 65–79, 106, 140–41, 170,
    201, 223
  allergies in, 61
  and cytokines, 218

and depression, 54
in epidemics, 14, 108, 183–84, 189
onset of CFIDS in, 74–76
symptoms in, 72, 79
Chills, 36
Chromosomes, and retroviruses,
    221–22
Chronic Epstein-Barr virus (CEBV),
    7, 106
*Chronic Fatigue and the Yeast
    Connection*, 95
Chronic fatigue/immune dysfunction
    syndrome (CFIDS), 8
  course of, 25–49
  and cytokine/retroviral theory,
    217–29
  definition of, 26
  and immune system, 93–103
  medication for, 157–68
  pre-existence of, 29
  prognosis of, 135–44
  theories about, 195–213
  treatment of, 145–55
  See also Diagnosis of CFIDS;
    Symptoms of CFIDS
Chronic fatigue syndrome (CFS), 7,
    188
Chronic infection, 224–25
Chronic metabolic myopathy, 210–11
Chronic mononucleosis, 106
  See also Mononucleosis
Clomipramine, 165
Clonazepam, 162, 165
Co-enzyme Q10, 175
Cognitive problems, 42, 43, 225
  in children, 76–78
  testing for, 112
  treatment of, 167
Common end pathway, 205, 206
Complete Blood Count (CBC), 85
Concentration, 42–43, 44–45, 73, 77
Congestion, 161–62
Constipation, 35
Coxsackie virus, 31, 116, 187, 203, 211
Cranial nerves, 42
Crook, William, 95
CT scan, 10, 91

Cure for CFIDS, 136, 145
Cyclic antidepressants, 165, 168
Cyclobenzaprine, 165
Cylert, 174
Cystic fibrosis, 20
Cytokines, 100, 112, 207, 209–10, 213, 215–19, 228
  as cause of depression, 58

Dairy products, 154
Definition of CFIDS, 72
DeFreitas, Elaine, 226–27, 229
Dementia, 45, 112, 225
Demitrack, M.A., 115
Depression, 12, 52–55, 115–16, 138, 208
  biologic, 57–58
  and immune system, 93
  primary, 54–55, 152, 163
  secondary, 55
  treatment of, 163–64, 166
Dermatographism, 39
Dermatomyositis, 173
Despair, 231
Diagnosis of CFIDS, 12–13, 51, 120, 148–49
  changes in, 19
  in children, 74, 75
  criteria for, 26–28, 137
  and evaluation, 83, 84, 86
  and immune system, 93
  by neurologists, 43, 45
  and pattern of symptoms, 25, 32
Diamox, 168
Diarrhea, 35
Diet, 153–54
Diphenhydramine, 161–62
Disability, 84
  measurement of, 119–21
  scale for, 122–24
Disability analyst, 121, 122
Disability benefits, 119
Dizziness, 32, 34, 42–43, 45, 73, 114, 138
DNA, 221–22, 224
Doxepin, 163–64

Drugs, 58, 155
Dysthymic disorder, 55

Ears, 40
  ringing in, 45
  testing of, 114
Economics of CFIDS, 14, 19, 83, 151
Education about CFIDS, 148–49, 150
Efamol, 175
Electromyography (EMG), 46
Electron micrograph, 114–15
Emotional disorders, 52–53, 78–79, 207–8
  cause of, 57–58
  misdiagnosis of, 73
Emotional stress, 31
Encephalitis, 208–9
Enteroviruses, 109, 203
Environmental illness, 212
Epidemics, 14, 137, 139–40, 181–94, 199, 202
  Adelaide, Australia, 184
  Akureyri, Iceland, 14, 137, 183–84
  Alaska, 137
  Ayrshire, Scotland, 187
  cause of, 14, 223
  comparing of, 137
  Great Ormond Street, London, 186–87
  Incline Village, Nevada, 13
  Lake Tahoe, 187–88
  Los Angeles, 137, 182–84
  Lyndonville, New York, 108, 139–40, 188–93, 198
  New York State, 184–85
  Punta Gorda, Florida, 137
  Royal Free Hospital, London, 137, 185–86
  Washington, D.C., 185
Epstein-Barr virus, 7, 17, 31, 52, 105–10, 170–71, 187, 203, 226
  and antibodies, 107–9
  and reactivation, 94–95, 95
  testing for, 83
  as trigger agent, 109–10
Etiologic testing, 84
Evening primrose oil, 175

Exclusionary tests, 84, 85–88
Exercise, 55, 116, 149, 152–53
Exhaustion, 47, 49
Eyes, 39–40
  pain in, 36

Fainting, 45
Family, 151, 199, 202
  and emotional disorders, 78
  in epidemics, 190
  support from, 154–55, 166
Fatality of CFIDS, 18, 136, 137–38,
  202, 223, 231
Fatigue, 9, 32, 33, 43, 46–47, 51, 75,
  76, 77–78
  cause of, 209
  and depression, 55
  testing for, 84, 87–88, 89, 114–15,
  116–17
  treatment of, 160, 162, 164–66
Febricula, 181
Fever, 36
  and immune system, 216
Fibromyalgia, 7, 36, 48–49, 63, 155,
  209
Fibrositis, 36
Flexeril, 165
Flu, 215–17, 224
Fluctuations, 32–33, 143
Fluoxetine, 164, 166, 168
Flushing, 48
Food and Drug Administration
  (FDA), 171
Food sensitivities, 154
Fractures, 47
Friends, support from, 154–55, 166
Functional capacity, 119

Gamma globulin, 147, 172–73
Gastric parietal cells, 99
Gender, 202
  in epidemics, 14
Generalists, 10
Genetics, 60–61, 221, 226–28, 232
  and cause of CFIDS, 205
Genitalia, 41
GI series, 89–90

Global frequency of CFIDS, 14
Glomerulonephritis, 17
Goiter, 39
Great Britain, research in, 203, 211
Great Ormond Street, London,
  outbreak in, 186–87
Groin, 41
Grufferman, Seymour, 93

Halcion, 162
Hay fever, 60
Headaches, 10, 32, 34, 42–43, 75
  and immune system, 216
  testing for, 91
  treatment of, 89, 160, 165, 167–68
Heart, 37, 41, 48
Heart murmur, 39, 41
Hemolytic anemia, 212
Hepatitis, 86
Herbal remedies, 148
Herman, Dr., 174
Herpes, 106, 109, 170–71, 203, 226
  and reactivation, 94–95
Histamine, 17
Hives, 48, 61
HIV virus, 18, 87, 199, 224
  and retrovirus, 222
Holmes, Michael, 126, 226
Hopelessness, 54, 55
Hormones, 207, 208–9
Hospital for Sick Children, outbreak
  in, 186–87
Hotchin, 205
HTLV-1 and HTLV-2, 222, 227–28
Huang and Quinlan method, 125
Human herpes virus, 203
Hyperimmunity, 99
Hyperplasia, 90
Hypersensitivity, 96
Hypersomnolence, 34
Hyperventilation, 167
Hypochondriasis, 48
Hypothyroidism, 207

Iceland. *See* Akureyri, Iceland,
  outbreak in
Immune complexes, 100

Immune reaction model, 17–18
Immune system, 17, 79, 93–103, 106
  activation of, 97–102
  and allergies, 60, 61
  and autoimmunity, 98–99
  and chemical sensitivities, 62
  and cytokines, 217–20
  and depression, 55
  dysfunction of, 94, 202, 209–10,
    225
  and retrovirus, 220–29, 224–25
  testing of, 83, 84, 90
  treatment of, 173–74
  workings of, 215–17
Immune system suppression, 94
Immunizations, 31
Immunoglobulin, 95–96, 225–26
Immunomodulatory drugs, 173–74
Impairment, 78
Inactivity, 75, 208
Incline Village, Nevada, outbreak in,
  13, 52, 105, 106–7, 112, 226
Inderal, 167
Infection, 94, 147, 170, 206, 211
  and allergies, 60
  and cytokines, 217–20
  and retrovirus, 222, 224–25, 226
  testing for, 88
Infection stimulated autoimmunity,
  206
Infectious diseases, 15, 232
  model of, 16
Infectious mononucleosis. *See*
  Mononucleosis
Influenza, 215
Injury, 31, 47, 56
Insidious onset
  in children, 74, 75–76, 77
Insomnia, 34, 164
  treatment of, 165–66
Insurance, 83
Interferon, 102, 112, 219, 228
Interleukin-2, 58, 100–1, 228
  and cancer, 218
  side effects of, 218–19
Interstitial cystitis, 46
Involuntary movements, 46

Jessop, Carol, 95
Joint pain, 32, 35, 47, 75
  treatment of, 160, 165
Jones, J.J., 105

Karnofsky Rating Scale, 124
Ketorolac, 165
Killer cells, 96–97
Kilocalorie Expenditure, 125
Klimas, Nancy, 103
Klonopin, 162
Komaroff, A., 226
Kutapressin, 174

Laboratory evaluation, 83–91
  cost of, 83–84
Labrinthitis, 45
Lake Tahoe, outbreak in, 52, 187–88
Lawsuits, 19
Leukemia, 90, 222
Lifestyle
  adjustment to, 149–51
  and disposition to CFIDS, 14, 135,
    136
Light-headedness, 48, 138
Light sensitivity, 36, 39
Limitations of CFIDS, 149–51
Listeriosis, 204
Liver, 39, 41, 42, 86, 161
  testing of, 90
London, outbreak in, 185–87
  See also Great Ormond Street,
    London; Royal Free Hospital,
    London
Los Angeles, outbreak in, 137,
  182–83, 199
Lumbar puncture, 89
Lupus erythematosis, 14, 17, 63, 88,
  99
Lyme disease, 88, 204
Lymph nodes, 32, 40–41, 42
  pain in, 35, 47, 51, 160
  testing of, 90
Lymphocytes, 96–97, 99–100, 116, 217
Lymphoma, 105–6, 222
Lyndonville, New York, outbreak in,
  108, 139–40, 188–93, 198

Magnesium, 115, 175
Magnetic resonance imaging (MRI),
    49, 91, 113
Malaise, 165–66
Malingering, 8, 53, 56–57, 138
Malpractice, 19
Mass hysteria, 54
Measles vaccine, 109
Mechanical damage model, 15–16
Medical history of patient, 25
Medical insurance. *See* Insurance
Medical technology, 19
Medication, 58, 145, 155, 157–68
    groups of, 159–60
    principles of, 157–59
Medicine and CFIDS, 18–21, 130–31
Meditation, 148, 151
Memory, 43, 44, 77, 164
    in testing, 112
Memory loss, 73
Mental illness, 53, 58, 208
    See also Depression
Mental state, 42
Metabolic myopathy, 210–11
Milk, 190–91
Mitochondria, 47, 117, 210–11
Mitogens, 97
Mitral valve prolapse, 37
Monoamine oxidase inhibitors, 164
Mononucleosis, 7, 17, 31, 49, 90, 106,
    109, 189, 205
    and Epstein-Barr virus, 105
Mouth ulcers, 35, 40
Multiple disease model, 196–98
Multiple sclerosis, 17, 43, 46, 51–52,
    111, 113, 122, 166, 222
    testing for, 89
Murdoch, J.C, 226
Muscle biopsies, 211
Muscles, 10, 42, 45–46, 63
    and immune system, 216
    pain in, 32, 36, 47, 160, 211
    testing of, 116–17
    treatment of, 165
Myalgia, 211
Myalgic encephalomyelitis (ME), 7,
    8, 187, 208

Naltrexone, 167
Narcolepsy, 114
Narcotics, 165
Nardil, 164
Nausea, 160, 216
Neck, 40
Nervous system, 42
Neurasthenia, 181
Neurologic symptoms, 32, 33–34,
    42–49, 73, 138, 142–43, 225
    examination for, 42, 113
    and retrovirus, 222
    treatment of, 160, 166
Neurology and CFIDS, 43, 45
Neuromyasthenia, 182
Neuropsychiatric symptoms, 33–34
Neurotransmitters, 58, 59
New York State, outbreak in, 184–85
    See also Lyndonville, New York
Night sweats, 36
Nonmedication treatments, 148
Nonsteroidal antiinflammatory drugs
    (NSAIDs), 161, 165, 168
Numbness, 34, 45–46
Nutritional supplements, 153–54,
    176–77

Onset of CFIDS, 28–31, 138–41, 199,
    202
    in children, 74–76, 170
    and cytokines, 217–18
Oral candidiasis. *See* Thrush
Organic brain syndrome, 53, 58
Organic depression, 58
Organic illnesses, 57
Osler, Sir William, 13
Oxygen, 114–15, 211

Pain, 47–49
    as cause of depression, 55
    perception of, 48
    treatment of, 165
Palpitations, 37, 48
    treatment of, 167
Panic, 48
    treatment of, 162, 167
Paresis, 185

Paresthesias, 34, 45-46
Patient
    history of, 25, 38
    and involvement in treatment, 146, 157
Pattern of symptoms. *See* Symptoms, pattern of
Pemoline, 174
Peterson, Daniel, 105, 171, 187, 226
Petit mal seizures, 73-74
Pharmacologic treatment, 155
Pharyngitis, 40
Phenelzine, 164
Photophobia, 36, 39
Physical examination, 38-39
Physician
    and acceptance of CFIDS, 12, 15, 18, 111, 138, 141
    and approach to CFIDS, 25-26
    and disability assessment, 120-21
    support from, 154-55, 166
Physiotherapy, 155
Placebo, 146-47
Pneumoccal vaccine, 96
Poisonings, 58
Polio, 195, 203
Poliomyelitis, 182, 183, 184, 185, 187
Pollen, 17, 60, 61, 98
Poly I-poly C, 171-72
Polymerase chain reaction (PCR), 227
Post-viral fatigue syndrome (PVFS), 7, 203
Precipitating event. *See* Trigger agent
Primary depression, 54-55, 115-16, 152, 163
Primary immunologic disorder, 209-10
Prodrome, 216, 217
Prognosis of CFIDS, 120, 135-44
    fatality, 137-38
    recovery, 138-43
Propranolol, 167
Provirus, 221
Prozac, 164, 166
Psychiatric illnesses, 57
Psychological testing, 112
Psychosomatic illness, 18, 30, 56, 111, 210

Psychotherapy, 155
Public knowledge of CFIDS, 20
Punta Gorda, Florida, outbreak in, 137

Radial plot of symptoms, 125-30
Rapid heartbeat, 167
Rash, 36-37, 39
Reactive arthritis, 205
Reading comprehension, 77
Recovery from CFIDS, 136, 138-43
Recurrence of CFIDS, 140
Red blood cell disorder, 211-12
Reduction of activity, 12, 27, 72, 122
Relapses, 32-33, 59, 138, 141-42, 150
Research into CFIDS, 49, 143, 162, 195-213, 231-32
    criteria for, 26-27
    funding for, 117-18, 233-34
Response to medication, 158
Retrovirus, 173, 204-5, 220-29
    treatment of, 226
Reverse transcriptase, 221, 226
Rheology, 211-12
Rheumatic fever, 17, 98, 206
Rheumatism, 39
Rheumatoid arthritis, 14, 63, 75, 87-88, 99, 160
Rheumatoid factor (RF), 87-88
RNA, 221-22
Royal Free Hospital, London, outbreak in, 52, 137, 185-86, 208

Sarcoidosis, 115
Scars, 47-48
School disorders, 73, 75, 76-78
Sclerotic plaques, 51
Sedimentation rate (sed rate), 86, 88
Seizures, 46, 73-74, 164
Serotonin uptake inhibitor, 164
Sertraline, 164
Severity of symptoms, 72, 202
    documentation of, 122, 126, 128
Shortness of breath, 37
Sickness impact profile, 125
Similarities of CFIDS with other illnesses, 51-63
Sinequan, 163-64

Single disease model, 196, 198–200
Sinusitis, 170
Sjogren's syndrome, 40
Skin, 39
Sleep apnea, 114, 165
Sleep disorder, 34
  improving, 151–52
  theory of, 209
  treatment of, 114, 162, 164–65
Social problems, 78–79
Social Security Administration, 131
Society for Epidemiologic Research, 190
Somatic symptoms, 73
Somatization, 56–57
Sore throat, 35, 75
Specialists, 9–10
SPECT scan, 49, 113
Spinal fluid, 208, 209
Spine, 45, 89
Spleen, 41, 42
  testing of, 90
Steinbach, Dr., 174
Steroids, 173
Stimulants, 174
Straus, S.E., 105
Stress, 31, 59, 109, 136, 151
Striae, 39
Suicide, 138, 231
Support for patients, 154–55, 166
Surgery, 31
Sweating, 48
Symptom clusters, 164–68
Symptoms of allergies, 15, 60–61
Symptoms of CFIDS, 12, 27, 32, 72, 79, 136, 140, 141, 202
  cause of, 174, 201
  in children, 72, 74, 75–76
  cognitive, 77–78
  and cytokines, 217–20
  description of, 33–38
  and disability, 122, 126, 128
  evaluation of, 84, 143
  fluctuation of, 158
  list of, 10–11
  neurological, 42–46
  onset of, 28–32

  pattern of, 8–13, 25–28, 54, 57, 59, 72, 85, 199
  psychosomatic, 56
  resolution of, 140–41
  treatment of, 145–47, 164–68
  worsening of, 147, 149–50, 151
  See also individual symptoms
Syncope, 138

T4 Lymphocyte, 222, 223, 225–26
Tapanui flu, 8
T-cell growth factor, 100
Teenagers, 141, 201
Temperature sensations, 36, 48
Tests for CFIDS, 19, 112–17
  See also Laboratory evaluation
Theories of CFIDS, 195–213
Throat, 40, 170
Thrush, 35, 40
Thyroid, 40, 87, 99, 207
Thyroiditis, 98–99, 207
Tingling, 34
Tobi, M., 105
Tolerance, 121
Tonsils, 40
Toradol, 165
Toxic encephalopathy, 31
Toxins, 58, 109
Toxoplasmosis, 204
Tranquilizers, 162
Treatment of CFIDS, 145–55
  future possibilities, 169–77
  types of, 148–55
Trexan, 167
Triazolam, 162
Trigger agent, 14, 15–16, 31–32, 191, 199, 205, 210, 224
  and cytokines, 218
  Epstein-Barr virus as, 109–10
  and interleukin-2, 101
  treatment of, 147–48
  as virus, 172
Tylenol, 160–61

Urine, 46
  testing of, 88

Vestibular studies, 114
Viral reactivation, 94–95
Virus, 30, 31, 60, 61, 215–16
  and antibodies, 98
  and immune system, 102
  and retrovirus, 221–22, 226
  testing of, 85
  theories of, 203–5
  treatment of, 172
  See also Epstein-Barr virus
Visualization, 148, 151
Visual/spatial perception, 77
Vitamin B12, 176
Vitamin C, 175–76
Vomiting, 35
Vulnerable state, 30

Washington, D.C., outbreak in, 185
Weight changes, 38, 154, 225
Wellbutrin, 164, 166
Word finding, 44–45, 77

X ray, 88

Yeast, 95, 204
  infection of, 40
  treatment of, 176
Yersinia enterocolitica, 191
Yoga, 148
"Yuppie flu," 7, 13, 52, 105

Zoloft, 164
Zovirax, 170–71